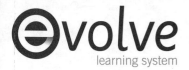
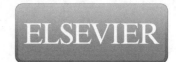
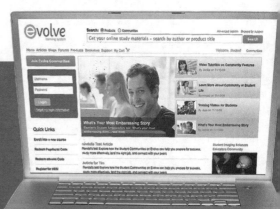

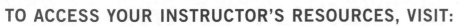

Workbook for Mosby's Respiratory Care Equipment

Ninth Edition

Laurie A. Freshwater, MA, RCP, RRT, RPFT
Health Sciences Division Director
Carteret Community College
Morehead City, North Carolina

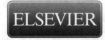

ELSEVIER
MOSBY

3251 Riverport Lane
Maryland Heights, Missouri 63043

WORKBOOK FOR MOSBY'S RESPIRATORY CARE EQUIPMENT   ISBN 978-0-323-09622-5

ISBN: 978-0323-09622-5

Content Strategy Director: Jeanne Olson
Content Manager: Billie Sharp
Senior Content Development Specialist: Kathleen Sartori
Publishing Services Manager: Hemamalini Rajendrababu
Project Manager: Antony Prince Dayalan

Printed in United States of America

Last digit is the print number: 9   8   7   6   5   4   3   2

To all my dedicated colleagues and friends in the
North Carolina Association of Respiratory Care Educators

"In the book of life, the answers aren't in the back."
Charles M. Schultz

Preface

The primary purpose of this workbook is to assist the respiratory care student in the comprehension of the material presented in the ninth edition of *Mosby's Respiratory Care Equipment*, by James Cairo.

Reading and studying from a textbook like this requires active involvement, because comprehension of this type does not occur automatically. In order for you to get as much out of your study time as possible, your reading must be a conscious, organized, active undertaking. An active reading session is made up of four separate stages: (1) previewing, (2) reading to organize, (3) reading to find significant facts, and (4) summarizing. The purpose of this workbook is to focus the reader on the learning objectives of the textbook. The learning objectives in this workbook that are tested on the NBRC CRT and RRT exams are referenced to the *Summary Content Outline for the CRT and Written RRT Examinations* (i.e. IA1). Try as much as possible to use your own words to answer the questions as this will help with summarizing what you have learned.

At the end of each chapter there are NBRC-type questions. These may be used as a self-assessment or by your instructor as an assignment. Think of this workbook as a scaffold to assist you in building the foundation of your professional knowledge.

All answers to the workbook can be found on Evolve: Evolve Resources for Cairo: Mosby's Respiratory Care Equipment, 9th edition: http://evolve.elsevier.com/Cairo/

Laurie A. Freshwater, MA, RCP, RRT, RPFT

*We wish to acknowledge Sindee Kalminson Karpel, MPA, RRT, the author of previous editions of this workbook.

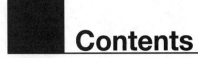

Contents

*Answers for the Workbook can be found on Evolve: **Evolve Resources for Cairo: Mosby's Respiratory Care Equipment, 9th edition:** http://evolve.elsevier.com/Cairo/

Basic Physics for the Respiratory Therapist

Upon completion of this chapter, you will be able to:

1. Differentiate between kinetic energy and potential energy.
2. Compare the physical and chemical properties of the three primary states of matter.
3. Explain why large amounts of energy are required to accomplish the changes associated with solid-liquid and liquid-gas phase transitions.
4. Convert temperature measurements from the Kelvin, Celsius, and Fahrenheit temperature scales.
5. Define *pressure*, and describe two devices that are commonly used to measure it.
6. List various pressure equivalents for 1 atm.
7. Calculate the density and specific gravity of liquids and gases.
8. Explain how changes in pressure, volume, temperature, and mass affect the behavior of an ideal gas.
9. Calculate the partial pressure of oxygen in a room air sample of gas obtained at 1 atm.
10. List the physical variables that influence the flow of a gas through a tube.
11. Explain how the pressure, velocity, and flow of a gas change as the gas moves from part of a tube with a large radius to another part with a small radius.
12. Describe the Venturi and Coanda effects and how both can be used in the design of respiratory care equipment.
13. State Ohm's law, and relate how changes in voltage and resistance affect current flow in a direct-current series circuit.
14. Describe three strategies that can be used to protect patients from electrical hazards.

"In physics, you don't have to go around making trouble for yourself — nature does it for you."
Frank Wilczek

ACHIEVING THE OBJECTIVES

1. Differentiate between kinetic energy and potential energy.

1A. Define kinetic energy.

_____

_____

1B. Define potential energy.

_____

_____

1C. List five common examples of kinetic energy.

_____

_____

_____

_____

_____

1D. List five common examples of potential energy.

_____

_____

_____

_____

_____

1E. As mass increases, potential energy and kinetic energy will

_____

_____.

1F. As velocity increases, kinetic energy will

_____

_____.

Think About This:

When a car is going downhill, why does the driver have to apply more pressure on the brakes to stop the car than if the car was moving on a level street?

2. Compare the physical and chemical properties of the three primary states of matter.

2A. List the three primary states of matter in order of greatest potential energy to least potential energy.

_____

_____

_____

2B. List the three primary states of matter in order of greatest kinetic energy to least kinetic energy.

_____

_____

_____

2C. The state of matter that possesses the weakest cohesive forces between constituent particles is

_____

_____.

2D. Why are gases and liquids described as fluids?

_____

_____

2E. The two states of matter that have no definite shape are

_____ and

_____.

2F. A state of matter that has no defined shape or volume and has no cohesive forces between constituent particles is a

_____.

2G. A state of matter that has weak intermolecular forces between constituent particles and is essentially incompressible is

_____.

2H. The two states of matter that have definite volume and cannot be compressed are

_____ and

_____.

2I. The one state of matter that has a definite shape and volume and cannot be compressed is a

_____.

2J. The one state of matter that has no definite shape and volume and can be compressed is a

_____.

Think About This:

Why won't gas stay in a cup?

Chapter **1** **Basic Physics for the Respiratory Therapist**

3. Explain why large amounts of energy are required to accomplish the changes associated with solid-liquid and liquid-gas phase transitions.

3A. Fill in the blanks in the following table.

Start from:	Change to:	Change of State:
Solid	Liquid	
Liquid	Solid	
Liquid	Gas	
Gas	Liquid	
Solid	Gas	

3B. The amount of heat that must be added to effect the change from a solid to liquid is called the

_____

_____.

3C. What effect does heat have on molecules?

_____

_____

3D. How does the application of heat to a liquid enhance the process of evaporation?

_____

_____

_____

_____

3E. Explain why the boiling point of water is lower at the Mount Washington Observatory in New Hampshire.

_____

_____

_____

3F. The state of matter at which water exists at temperatures between 0° C and 100° C is

_____.

3G. What happens to water at temperatures above 374° C?

_____

_____

3H. Describe the difference between a gas and a vapor.

_____

_____

_____

_____

Think About This:

Why is salt used to make ice cream?

4. Convert temperature measurements from the Kelvin, Celsius, and Fahrenheit temperature scales.

4A. Identify the two most common reference temperatures.

_____

_____

4B. Why is the Fahrenheit scale not a centigrade scale?

_____

_____

_____

4C. On which scale is absolute zero found?

_____

4D. Convert 25° C to Kelvin.

_____

4E. Convert 150° K to Celsius.

_____

4F. Convert 92° F to Kelvin.

_____

4G. Convert 100° K to Fahrenheit.

_____

_____

Think About This:

Why shouldn't thermometers be placed directly in the sun to measure air temperature?

5. Define _pressure_, and describe two devices that are commonly used to measure it.

5A. What is the definition of _gas pressure_?

_____

_____

5B. Why is the atmospheric pressure on Mount Washington less than that in New Orleans?

_____

_____

5C. Describe how a mercury barometer measures atmospheric pressure.

_____

_____

_____

5D. Describe how an aneroid barometer measures atmospheric pressure.

_____

_____

_____

Think About This:

Why will a potato chip bag packed and sealed in New Orleans burst open in Denver?

6. List various pressure equivalents for 1 atm.

6A. 1 atm = _____ psi

6B. 1 atm = _____ mm Hg

6C. 1 atm = _____ cm H$_2$O

6D. 1 atm = _____ kPa

Think About This:

What is happening inside the highs and lows on a weather map?

7. Calculate the density and specific gravity of liquids and gases.

7A. What is the formula for density?

_____

_____

7B. What are the units of expression for the density of a solid?

_____

_____

7C. What are the units of expression for the density of a gas?

_____

_____

7D. The volume in liters that 1 mole of gas occupies at standard temperature and pressure, dry (STPD) is

_____

_____

7E. Given that the mass of oxygen (molecular weight) is 32 g, calculate the density of oxygen.

_____

_____

7F. Given that the mass of nitrogen is 28 g, calculate the density of nitrogen.

_____

_____

7G. Given that the mass of helium is 4 g, calculate the density of helium.

_____

_____

7H. What are the values for STPD?

_____

_____

7I. A block of aluminum has a volume of 15.0 mL and weighs 40.5 g. What is its density?

_____

_____

7J. Note that 1.00 g of oxygen gas (O$_2$) has a volume of 670.2 mL. The same mass of carbon dioxide gas (CO$_2$) occupies 505.8 mL. What are the densities of the two gases?

_____

_____

7K. What is the reference substance used to calculate the specific gravity of a liquid?

_____

_____

7L. What is the difference between density and specific gravity?

_____

_____

7M. What does Avogadro's number represent?

_____

_____

7N. How is specific gravity calculated?

_____

_____

7O. If a liquid has a specific gravity of 1.21, is it lighter or heavier than water?

_____

_____

Think About This:

What does the specific gravity of urine tell us about the function of the kidneys?

8. Explain how changes in pressure, volume, temperature, and mass affect the behavior of an ideal gas.

Fill in the blanks in the following table.

	Law	Description	Formula
8A.	Boyle's law		
8B.		The volume of a given amount of gas held at a constant pressure increases proportionately with increases in the temperature of the gas.	
8C.			$P_1/T_1 = P_2/T_2$
8D.		Equal volumes of gas at the same pressure and temperature contain the same number of molecules.	
8E.			$PB = PO_2 + PN_2 + PCO_2 + P \text{ (trace gases)}$
8F.	Combined gas law		
8G.		When a gas is confined in a space adjacent to a liquid, a certain number of gas molecules dissolve in the liquid phase.	
8H.	Graham's law		
8I.			$\dot{V}gas = A \times D \times \Delta P/T$

8J. Helium takes up 5.71 L at 0° C and 3.95 atm. What is the volume of the same amount of helium at 32° F and 800 mm Hg? What gas law did you use to calculate the answer?

_____

_____

_____

_____

_____

8K. A 100 L sample of helium at 27° C is cooled at constant pressure to –55° C. Calculate the new volume of the helium. What gas law did you use in this situation?

_____

_____

_____

_____

_____

8L. If you were to take a volleyball SCUBA (self-contained underwater breathing apparatus) diving with you, what would be its new volume if it started at the surface with a volume of 2.5 L, under a pressure of 760 mm Hg, and with a temperature of 22° C? On your dive, you take it to a place where the pressure is 2943 mm Hg and the temperature is 0.25° C. What gas law did you use in this situation?

_____

_____

_____

_____

_____

8M. Name the four factors that play roles in the diffusion of oxygen across the alveolar capillary membrane.

_____

_____

_____

_____

_____

Think About This:

What happens to the volume of gas in a SCUBA diver's body cavities as the diver descends?

9. Calculate the partial pressure of oxygen in a room air sample of gas obtained at 1 atm.

9A. The air we breathe consists of what gases?

_____

_____

9B. List the gases contained in air and their percentage.

_____

_____

9C. How can total atmospheric pressure be calculated?

_____

_____

_____

9D. What is the formula to calculate the partial pressure of a gas (in mm Hg) in a sample of room air?

_____

_____

9E. Calculate the partial pressure of oxygen in a room air sample of gas obtained at 1 atm.

_____

_____

9F. What formula is used to calculate the partial pressure of inspired oxygen?

_____

_____

9G. Mount Rainier's Columbia Crest (its current summit), in Washington State, is 14,411 feet above sea level. The barometric pressure is 459 mm Hg. Calculate the partial pressure of inspired oxygen at body temperature and saturation.

_____

_____

9H. A mixture of neon and argon gases exerts a total pressure of 2.39 atm. The partial pressure of the neon alone is 1.84 atm; what is the partial pressure of the argon?

_____

_____

Think About This:

Why would an otherwise healthy visitor to Mesa Verde National Park, Colorado (6960 feet above sea level), be in the ranger station receiving supplemental oxygen for shortness of breath?

Chapter 1 Basic Physics for the Respiratory Therapist

10. List the physical variables that influence the flow of a gas through a tube.

10A. Identify the three patterns of flow in Figure 1-1.

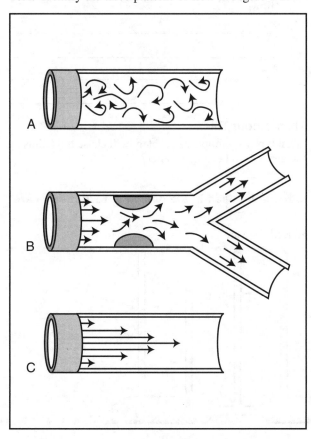

FIGURE 1-1

_____

_____

10B. Which of the flow patterns is normally associated with the movement of fluids through tubes with smooth surfaces and fixed radii?

_____

10C. The pressure required to produce a given flow is influenced more by the density of the fluid than by its viscosity when which flow pattern is present?

_____

10D. In the lung, where is flow predominantly laminar?

_____

_____

10E. In the lung, where is flow predominantly turbulent?

_____

_____

10F. In the lung, where is flow predominantly transitional?

_____

_____

Think About This:

Why is laminar flow an important factor in flight?

11. Explain how the pressure, velocity, and flow of a gas change as it moves from part of a tube with a large radius to another part with a small radius.

11A. What two factors must be considered when describing gas movement through a tube?

_____

_____

11B. According to Poiseuille, what factors determine the resistance to flow?

_____

_____

11C. Calculate the resistance to flow if the viscosity = 1, length = 1, and radius = 1.

_____

_____

11D. Calculate the resistance to flow if the viscosity = 1, length = 1, and radius = 0.5.

_____

_____

11E. Calculate the resistance to flow if the viscosity = 1, length = 1, and radius = 2.

_____

_____

11F. Calculate the resistance to flow if the viscosity = 2, length = 1, and radius = 1.

_____

_____

11G. Calculate the resistance to flow if the viscosity = 0.5, length = 1, and radius = 1.

_____

_____

11H. Calculate the resistance to flow if the viscosity = 1, length = 2, and radius = 1.

_____

_____

11I. Calculate the resistance to flow if the viscosity = 1, length = 0.5, and radius = 1.

_____

_____

11J. Using the previous seven calculations, determine which of the factors (viscosity, tube length, or tube radius) causes the greatest change in resistance to flow.

_____

_____

_____

_____

Think About This:

What type of pulmonary problem will cause the radius of the airways to become smaller?

12. Describe the Venturi and Coanda effects and how both can be used in the design of respiratory care equipment.

12A. Explain why the fourth manometer in Figure 1-2 shows reduced pressure.

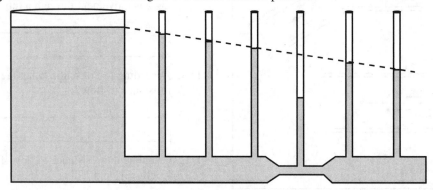

FIGURE 1-2
(Redrawn from Nave CR, Nave BC: *Physics for the health sciences*, ed 3, Philadelphia, 1985, Saunders.)

_____

_____

Questions 12B through 12D refer to Figure 1-3.

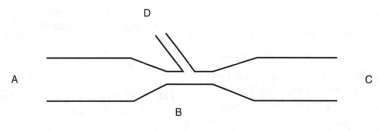

FIGURE 1-3

12B. As a gas moves from point *A* to point *C* in Figure 1-3, what happens to the speed of the gas as it flows through the constriction in the tube labeled *B*?

_____

_____

12C. As the gas passes through the constriction in the tube in Figure 1-3, what happens to the gas around point *D* in this figure?

_____

_____

12D. What happens to the speed of the gas as it emerges from the constriction in the tube in Figure 1-3 and flows toward point *C* in this figure?

_____

_____

Questions 12E through 12G refer to Figure 1-4.

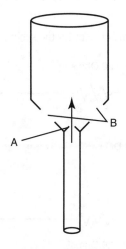

FIGURE 1-4

12E. What happens to the velocity of a gas as it flows through point *A* in Figure 1-4?

_____

_____

12F. What happens to the pressure as the gas flows through point *A* in Figure 1-4?

_____

_____

12G. What will happen to air just outside the "ports" labeled *B* in Figure 1-4 as a gas is going through the constriction labeled *A*?

_____

_____

12H. List three respiratory care devices that utilize the Venturi principle.

_____

_____

_____

12I. The Coanda effect will cause the water from the faucet to travel toward which direction (Figure 1-5) — *A, B,* or *C* — after it touches the back of the spoon?

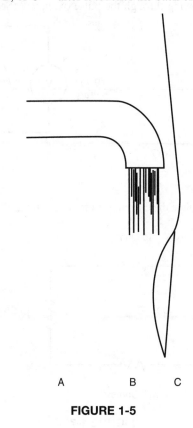

A   B   C

FIGURE 1-5

_____

_____

12J. What type of respiratory care device uses the Coanda effect?

_____

_____

Think About This:
Which principle helps airplanes lift off the ground?

Chapter **1** **Basic Physics for the Respiratory Therapist**

13. **State Ohm's law, and relate how changes in voltage and resistance affect current flow in a direct-current series circuit.**

13A. Name the three factors involved in Ohm's law.

_____

_____

13B. What is the formula for Ohm's law?

_____

13C. A 9-volt (9 V) battery supplies power to a pulse oximeter with a resistance (R) of 18 ohms (Ω). How much current is flowing through the pulse oximeter? (See Figure 1-6.)

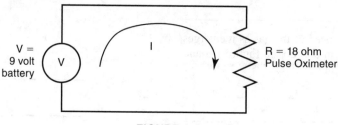

FIGURE 1-6

13D. Calculate the current for the schematic in Figure 1-7.

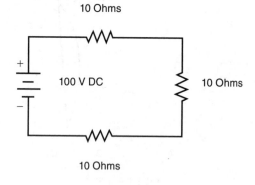

FIGURE 1-7

13E. Calculate the current for the schematic in Figure 1-8.

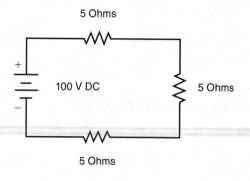

FIGURE 1-8

13F. Calculate the current for the schematic in Figure 1-9.

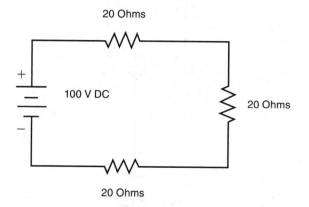

FIGURE 1-9

13G. What happens to the current flow in a direct-current series circuit when voltage remains constant and resistance increases?

_____

_____

13H. What happens to the current flow in a direct-current series circuit when resistance remains constant and the voltage is increased?

_____

_____

13I. Calculate the current in a direct-current parallel circuit when the voltage is 120 and $R_1 = 30$, $R_2 = 60$, $R_3 = 30$, and $R_4 = 20$ Ω.

_____

_____

_____

_____

Think About This:

Will a 1.5 V direct-current (DC) circuit with one light bulb be brighter than a 3 V DC circuit with two light bulbs in series?

14. Describe three strategies that can be used to protect patients from electrical hazards.

14A. Describe how grounding offers protection from electrical hazards.

_____

_____

_____

_____

14B. How do ground-fault circuit interrupters protect against electrical hazards?

_____

_____

_____

14C. What is the purpose of regular inspection of respiratory equipment by a hospital's biomedical equipment department?

_____

_____

_____

_____

Think About This:

Why is static electricity build-up hazardous in an operating room?

Name _____

Date _____

NATIONAL BOARD FOR RESPIRATORY CARE (NBRC)–TYPE QUESTIONS

1. Another name for *supercooled liquids* is which of the following?
   A. *Elements*
   B. *Compounds*
   C. *Crystalline solids*
   D. *Amorphous solids*

2. The melting of ice demonstrates which of the following?
   A. An increase in potential energy
   B. An increase in kinetic energy
   C. The latent heat of fusion
   D. The process of sublimation

3. The opposite of evaporation is which of the following?
   A. Respiration
   B. Vaporization
   C. Condensation
   D. Sublimation

4. A sample of gas expands isothermally from 10.0 L to 30.0 L. If the initial pressure was 1140 mm Hg, what is the new pressure?
   A. 3420 mm Hg
   B. 380 mm Hg
   C. 127 mm Hg
   D. 760 mm Hg

5. A sample of gas initially occupies 3.0 mL at a pressure of 47.8 mm Hg. The pressure is increased to 746 mm Hg. What is the new volume?
   A. 0.192 mL
   B. 46.8 mL
   C. 0.0214 mL
   D. 5.21 mL

6. A gas system has an initial temperature of 142° C with the volume unknown. When the temperature changes to 46.20° K, the volume is found to be 1.58 L. What was the initial volume in liters (L)?
   A. 2.05 L
   B. 4.9 L
   C. 10.8 L
   D. 14.2 L

7. Under the same conditions of temperature and pressure, a liquid differs from a gas because the particles of the liquid
   A. Are in a constant straight-line motion.
   B. Take the shape of the container they occupy.
   C. Have no regular arrangement.
   D. Have stronger forces of attraction between them.

8. The volume of a given mass of an ideal gas at constant pressure is which of the following?
   A. Directly proportional to the Kelvin temperature
   B. Directly proportional to the Celsius temperature
   C. Inversely proportional to the Kelvin temperature
   D. Inversely proportional to the Celsius temperature

9. A mixture of helium and oxygen exerts a combined pressure of 6 atm, and the partial pressure of oxygen is 4 atm. What is the partial pressure of helium?
   A. 1520 mm Hg
   B. Not enough information
   C. 6600 mm Hg
   D. 7600 mm Hg

10. A cylinder contains helium and oxygen and exerts a total pressure of 7.00 atm. The cylinder has 42.8% helium. What is the partial pressure of oxygen in this cylinder?
    A. 435 mm Hg
    B. 2277 mm Hg
    C. 3043 mm Hg
    D. 4004 mm Hg

11. Calculate the total current through the circuit in Figure 1-10.

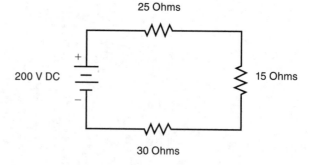

FIGURE 1-10

    A. 0.35 A
    B. 2.86 A
    C. 3.50 A
    D. 28 A

12. According to Fick's first law of diffusion, flow of gas across a semipermeable membrane will be reduced when which of the following occurs?
    A. Surface area increases
    B. Wall thickness increases
    C. Wall thickness decreases
    D. Gas diffusivity increases

2 Principles of Infection Control

Upon completion of this chapter, you will be able to:
1. Identify the major groups of microorganisms associated with nosocomial pneumonia.
2. List four factors that can influence the effectiveness of a germicide.
3. Define *high-level disinfection, intermediate-level disinfection,* and *low-level disinfection.*
4. Describe the process of pasteurization and its application to the disinfection of respiratory care equipment.
5. Explain how quaternary ammonium compounds (quats), alcohols, acetic acid, phenols, glutaraldehyde, hydrogen peroxide, and iodophors and other halogenated compounds are used as disinfectants.
6. Name the four physical methods commonly used to sterilize medical devices.
7. Discuss the principle of ethylene oxide sterilization.
8. Identify infection risk devices used in respiratory care.
9. Describe three components of an effective infection surveillance program.
10. Compare standard precautions with transmission-based precautions.
11. List the agents most commonly associated with febrile respiratory illnesses that are potential causes of mass casualty events.

"No science is immune to the infection of politics and the corruption of power."
Jacob Bronowski

13

1. Identify the major groups of microorganisms associated with nosocomial pneumonia.

1A. Identify the bacteria in Figure 2-1.

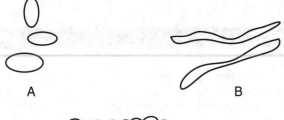

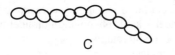

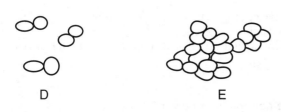

FIGURE 2-1

A. _____

B. _____

C. _____

D. _____

E. _____

1B. What is the size range for bacteria?

_____

_____

1C. How are bacteria generally classified?

_____

_____

1D. List five bacteria that will appear blue or violet following a Gram stain.

_____

_____

_____

_____

1E. List nine gram-negative pathogens.

_____

_____

_____

_____

_____

_____

_____

_____

_____

_____

1F. What stains are used to identify *Mycobacterium*?

_____

_____

1G. Within what temperature range do pathogenic organisms typically grow?

_____

_____

1H. Why are bacteria that produce endospores a constant source of concern for infection control personnel?

_____

_____

_____

_____

1I. The two most notable sources of bacterial endospores are

_____ and

_____.

1J. Which species of bacteria are gram-positive aerobes?

_____

_____

_____

_____

1K. Which species of bacteria are gram-negative aerobes?

_____

_____

_____

_____

_____

_____

1L. What is the size range for viruses?

_____

_____

1M. Name three ways that viruses are classified.

_____

_____

_____

1N. List four viruses that can cause pneumonia.

_____

_____

_____

_____

1O. Which virus causes severe acute respiratory syndrome?

_____

_____

1P. Which organism causes typhus, Rocky Mountain spotted fever, and Q fever?

_____

_____

1Q. The intracellular parasite that is associated with pneumonia, sinusitis, pharyngitis, and bronchiolitis is

_____

_____.

1R. List three examples of protozoan infections.

_____

_____

_____

1S. Three fungi that cause opportunistic infections are

_____,

_____, and

_____.

1T. Name three gram-negative bacteria commonly associated with ventilator-associated pneumonia.

_____

_____

1U. Name two gram-positive bacteria commonly associated with ventilator-associated pneumonia.

_____

_____

1V. Name the four routes of transmissions for infectious particles.

_____

_____

1W. Define the term *fomite*.

_____

_____

1X. Complete the following table.

Disease-Causing Organism	Route of Transmission
Legionella pneumophila	
Mycobacterium tuberculosis	
Streptococcus pneumoniae	
Pseudomonas aeruginosa	
Staphylococcus aureus	

1Y. Why are patients with endotracheal tubes, surgical wounds, intravenous catheters, Foley catheters, and burns at risk for developing nosocomial infections?

_____

_____

_____

_____

Think About This:
How do "super bacteria" develop?

2. List four factors that can influence the effectiveness of a germicide. (IIB1)

2A. Define the term *germicide*.

_____

_____

2B. How do these agents destroy the pathogenic microorganisms?

_____

_____

2C. What is the difference between a germicide and a disinfectant?

_____

_____

_____

_____

_____

_____

2D. The elimination of all forms of microbial life is called

_____

_____.

2E. How do the number and location of microorganisms affect the ability of a germicide to work?

_____

_____

_____

_____

_____

2F. Name the microbe that is most resistant to disinfection and sterilization.

_____

_____

2G. As a disinfectant's concentration increases, what happens to its potency?

_____

_____

2H. Which gram-negative aerobic organism shows greater resistance to some disinfectants?

_____

_____

_____

2I. Increasing the temperature of a germicide will ____ _____ its activity.

2J. Which two types of disinfectants increase antimicrobial activity when the pH is increased?

_____

_____

2K. Which three types of disinfectants decrease antimicrobial activity when the pH is increased?

_____

_____

_____

2L. Relative humidity will affect the disinfectant activity of which gaseous disinfectants?

_____

_____

2M. What is the first step in the decontamination process?

_____

_____

Think About This:

What other industries use germicides?

3. Define *high-level disinfection*, *intermediate-level disinfection*, and *low-level disinfection*. (IIB1)

3A. How does disinfection differ from sterilization?

_____

_____

3B. What is a disinfectant that can eliminate spores called?

_____

_____

3C. Define *high-level disinfection*.

_____

_____

_____

3D. How does intermediate-level disinfection differ from high-level disinfection?

_____

_____

3E. What are low-level disinfectants?

_____

_____

Think About This:

Why should germicides be used in the cleaning of equipment used for tattooing, ear-piercing and body-piercing, acupuncture, and hair removal by electrolysis?

4. Describe the process of pasteurization and its application to the disinfection of respiratory care equipment. (IIB1)

4A. What happens to cell proteins during pasteurization?

_____

_____

4B. Describe flash process pasteurization.

_____

_____

4C. What is flash process pasteurization usually used for?

_____

_____

4D. Describe batch process pasteurization.

_____

_____

4E. Why is batch process pasteurization used with respiratory care equipment?

_____

_____

_____

_____

_____

Think About This:

In addition to milk, what foods and liquids are pasteurized?

5. Explain how quaternary ammonium compounds (quats), alcohols, acetic acid, phenols, glutaraldehyde, hydrogen peroxide, and iodophors and other halogenated compounds are used as disinfectants. (IIB1)

5A. What is the mode of action for disinfection by quats?

_____

_____

_____

_____

5B. What germicidal properties do quaternary ammonium compounds have?

_____

_____

5C. What are quats used for in the hospital?

_____

_____

5D. What germicidal properties do ethyl and isopropyl alcohol have?

_____

_____

5E. What is the mode of action for disinfection by alcohols?

_____

_____

5F. According to the Centers for Disease Control and Prevention (CDC), what exposure time should be used with alcohol?

_____

_____

5G. What are alcohols used to disinfect in the hospital?

_____

_____

_____

_____

5H. What germicidal properties does acetic acid have?

_____

_____

5I. What is the mode of action for disinfection by acetic acid?

_____

_____

17

5J. What is the optimum concentration of acetic acid for disinfection use?

_____

_____

5K. Why is acetic acid useful in decontaminating home care respiratory equipment?

_____

_____

_____

_____

5L. What germicidal properties do phenols have?

_____

_____

5M. What is the mode of action for disinfection by phenols?

_____

_____

5N. What are phenols used to disinfect in the hospital?

_____

_____

5O. What germicidal properties do iodophors have?

_____

_____

5P. What is the mode of action for disinfection by iodophors?

_____

_____

5Q. What are iodophors used for in the hospital?

_____

_____

5R. What disinfecting agent is recommended by the CDC to clean blood spills?

_____

_____

5S. What germicidal properties does glutaraldehyde have?

_____

_____

5T. What is the mode of action for disinfection by glutaraldehyde?

_____

_____

5U. Compare acid and alkaline glutaraldehyde.

	Acid Glutaraldehyde	Alkaline Glutaraldehyde
Activation		
pH		
Germicidal properties		
Exposure		
Shelf-life		

5V. What germicidal properties does hydrogen peroxide have?

_____

_____

5W. What is the mode of action for disinfection by hydrogen peroxide?

_____

_____

_____

5X. How can hydrogen peroxide be a sterilizing agent?

_____

_____

Think About This:

How do you clean your kitchen and bathrooms?

6. Name the four physical methods commonly used to sterilize medical devices. (IIB1)

6A. List the four physical methods commonly used to sterilize medical devices.

_____

_____

_____

_____

6B. Which physical method is used to sterilize contaminated disposable equipment?

_____

_____

6C. Which physical method is used to sterilize laboratory glassware and surgical instruments?

_____

_____

6D. Which physical method of sterilization has questionable effectiveness against spores?

_____

_____

6E. Which physical method of sterilization is highly effective, is inexpensive, creates no air pollution, and is the most versatile?

_____

_____

6F. How does an autoclave increase the temperature of steam above 100° C?

_____

_____

_____

_____

6G. How long does contaminated equipment need to be autoclaved to be sterilized at 121° C and at 132° C?

_____

_____

6H. What is done to ensure the quality control of the autoclaving process?

_____

_____

_____

_____

_____

Think About This:

Why should disposable equipment not be reused?

7. Discuss the principle of ethylene oxide sterilization. (IIB1)

7A. Describe the properties of ethylene oxide (ETO).

_____

_____

7B. What is the mode of action for ETO as a sterilant?

_____

_____

7C. Upon what does the effectiveness of ETO depend?

_____

_____

_____

_____

_____

_____

7D. What two factors can decrease sterilization time?

_____

_____

7E. The materials that can be used to package equipment for ETO sterilization are

_____

_____.

7F. List the stages of automated ETO sterilization.

_____

_____

_____

_____

_____

7G. What conditions are necessary for the mechanical aeration of equipment that is sterilized with ETO?

_____

_____

7H. Why is aeration of ETO-sterilized equipment at room temperature dangerous?

_____

_____

7I. How is the effectiveness of ETO sterilization monitored?

_____

_____

_____

7J. What is the Occupational Safety & Health Administration (OSHA) standard for ETO exposure?

_____

_____

Think About This:

What type of protective equipment should be worn when working with ETO?

8. Identify infection risk devices used in respiratory care. (IIB1)

8A. What are the three categories described by Spaulding for stratifying the risk of infection from reusable patient care equipment?

_____

_____

_____

8B. Give examples of equipment in each of the risk-infection categories, and explain why they are included there.

Category	Types of Equipment	Reason for Category

8C. Why is sterility not necessary with equipment that comes in contact with only the skin?

_____

_____

8D. What method(s) of processing is/are recommended for respiratory care equipment?

_____

_____

8E. If the aforementioned processing (in question 8D) is not feasible, what should be done?

_____

_____

8F. What setup should be used to monitor an intubated patient with a respirometer?

_____

_____

8G. Describe the recommended steps for processing bronchoscopes.

_____

_____

_____

_____

8H. What are the recommendations for changing or replacing large-volume jet nebulizers and medication nebulizers and their reservoirs and tubing?

_____

_____

8I. How should water in a ventilator circuit or nebulizer tubing be disposed of?

_____

_____

8J. Give examples of methods to reduce the risk of nosocomial pneumonia in mechanically ventilated patients.

_____

_____

_____

Think About This:

How is soiled linen decontaminated in a hospital?

9. Describe three components of an effective infection surveillance program. (IIB1)

9A. What is the purpose of an infection surveillance program?

_____

_____

9B. Complete the following table.

	Surveillance Components	Description (Give Example)
1		
2		
3		

9C. Why is identifying the cause of nosocomial infections important?

_____

_____

Think About This:

How is respiratory care equipment in the home monitored for infection control?

10. Compare standard precautions with transmission-based precautions. (IIB5)

10A. When should standard precautions be used in the hospital?

_____

_____

10B. From what particular substances are standard precautions providing protection?

_____

_____

10C. What is the goal of standard precautions?

_____

_____

_____

10D. What needs to be done by the respiratory care practitioner to ensure standard precautions are followed?

_____

_____

10E. What is the goal of transmission-based precautions?

_____

_____

_____

_____

10F. When should transmission-based precautions be used in the hospital?

_____

_____

_____

_____

10G. When does hand-washing (hand hygiene) need to be performed?

_____

_____

_____

10H. When do gloves need to be worn?

_____

_____

_____

10I. When do gowns need to be worn?

_____

_____

_____

10J. When do face shields or masks with protective eyewear need to be worn?

_____

_____

_____

10K. What are the five components of respiratory hygiene/cough etiquette?

_____

_____

_____

_____

_____

10L. What are the main components of safe injection practices?

_____

_____

_____

_____

10M. Complete the following table.

Precaution Type	Pathogen Known/Suspected or Procedure	Precautions
Airborne precautions		
Droplet precautions		
Contact precautions		

Think About This:

How often do you wash your hands when caring for a sick family member or friend?

11. List the agents most commonly associated with febrile respiratory illnesses that are potential causes of mass casualty events. (IIB4)

11A. What does an effective disaster infection control plan include?

_____

_____

_____

_____

11B. Name two intentional causes of febrile respiratory illness (FRI) that can lead to a mass casualty event.

_____

_____

11C. Name five contagious causes of FRI that can lead to a mass casualty event.

_____

_____

_____

_____

11D. Which biological agents are transmitted person-to-person through the inhalation of droplets or aerosol?

_____

_____

11E. Airborne infection isolation placement is recommended for use with patients infected with which three biological agents?

_____

_____

_____

Think About This:

I was vaccinated against smallpox before 1980; am I still protected?

NATIONAL BOARD FOR RESPIRATORY CARE (NBRC)–TYPE QUESTIONS

1. A sputum specimen is received in the lab. A smear is made, and the specimen is subjected to Gram staining. A microscopic examination reveals spherical purple-staining clusters. Which of the following characteristics can reasonably be assumed about this organism?
   1. Gram-negative
   2. In the bacilli family
   3. In the streptococci family
   4. Associated with causing pneumonia
      A. 1, 2, and 3 only
      B. 1, 3, and 4 only
      C. 2 and 3 only
      D. 4 only

2. Which of the following statements are true about the amount of time required to kill microorganisms?
   1. The time decreases as the strength of the germicide increases.
   2. The time is directly proportional to the number of pathogens.
   3. The time increases as the microbial population increases.
   4. Time varies with the resistance of the organism.
      A. 2, 3, and 4 only
      B. 3 and 4 only
      C. 1 and 3 only
      D. 2 and 3 only

3. The medical disorder that increases patient susceptibility to nosocomial infection include which of the following?
   A. Hypoglycemia
   B. Altered B cells
   C. Hyperbilirubinemia
   D. Hypogammaglobulinemia

4. Bacterial spores can be inactivated by exposure to which of the following?
   A. 10 hours of iodophors
   B. 8 hours of glutaraldehyde
   C. 30 minutes of isopropyl alcohol
   D. 6 hours of quaternary ammonium compounds

5. The household item that is useful for disinfection of respiratory home care equipment is which of the following?
   A. Peroxide
   B. Vinegar
   C. Bleach
   D. Lye

6. At high altitudes, sterilization by boiling must be prolonged primarily because of which of the following?
   A. Increased oxygen content
   B. Reduced oxygen content
   C. Increased normal boiling point
   D. Reduced normal boiling point

7. Which of the following viruses will cause bronchiolitis?
   A. Influenza
   B. Rhinovirus
   C. Herpes zoster
   D. Respiratory syncytial

8. Hepatitis B is spread by which type of transmission?
   A. Droplet nuclei
   B. Airborne
   C. Direct contact
   D. Food-borne vehicle

9. A highly effective, versatile, and inexpensive method of sterilization consists of the use of which of the following?
   A. Phenols
   B. Alcohol
   C. Autoclaving
   D. Ethylene oxide

10. A patient arrives in the emergency department with a history of increasing dyspnea on exertion, weight loss, and a positive cough history. The physician suspects tuberculosis. The most appropriate type of precaution to use for this patient is which of the following?
    A. Contact precautions
    B. Standard precautions
    C. Droplet precautions
    D. Airborne precautions

Manufacture, Storage, and Transport of Medical Gases

LEARNING OBJECTIVES

Upon completion of this chapter, you will be able to:
 1. Describe the chemical and physical properties of the medical gases most often encountered in respiratory care.
 2. Identify various types of medical gas cylinders (e.g., types 3, 3A, 3AA, and 3AL).
 3. Identify the following cylinder markings: Department of Transportation (DOT) specifications, service pressure, hydrostatic testing dates, manufacturer's identification, ownership mark, serial number, and cylinder size.
 4. List the color codes used to identify medical gas cylinders.
 5. Discuss United States Pharmacopeia (USP) purity standards for medical gases.
 6. Compare the operation of direct-acting cylinder valves with that of diaphragm-type cylinder valves.
 7. Explain American Standards Association (ASA) indexing, the Pin Index Safety System (PISS), and the Diameter Index Safety System (DISS).
 8. Identify and correct a problem with cylinder valve assembly.
 9. Calculate the gas volume remaining in a compressed-gas cylinder, and estimate the duration of gas flow based on the cylinder's gauge pressure.
10. Describe the components of a bulk liquid oxygen system, and discuss National Fire Protection Association (NFPA) recommendations for the storage and use of liquid oxygen in bulk systems.
11. Discuss the operation of a portable liquid oxygen system and describe NFPA recommendations for these systems.
12. Calculate the duration of a portable liquid oxygen supply.
13. Identify three types of medical air compressors, and describe the operational theory of each.
14. Summarize NFPA recommendations for medical air supply safety.
15. Compare continuous supply systems with alternating central supply systems.
16. Identify a DISS station outlet and a quick-connect station outlet.
17. Compare the operational theory of a membrane oxygenator with that of a molecular sieve oxygenator.

"Not all chemicals are bad. Without chemicals such as hydrogen and oxygen, for example, there would be no way to make water, a vital ingredient in beer."
Dave Barry

ACHIEVING THE OBJECTIVES

1. Describe the chemical and physical properties of the medical gases most often encountered in respiratory care. (IIA9a)

1A. The nonflammable substance that can exist as a liquid or a gas, is colorless, odorless, has a slightly acidic taste, and has a molecular weight of 44.01 and a critical temperature of 31.1° C is _____ _____ .

1B. The nonflammable gas that has a molecular weight of 4.00, is tasteless, and has a critical temperature of −267.0° C is _____ .

1C. _____ is a gas that is a powerful pulmonary vasodilator used to treat persistent pulmonary hypertension of the newborn.

1D. The nonflammable substance that can exist as a liquid or a gas, has a molecular weight of 44.01, and is used as an anesthetic is _____ .

1E. _____ is a colorless, odorless, tasteless, flammable gas that binds easily to hemoglobin.

1F. The nonflammable gas or liquid that supports combustion, has a critical temperature of −118.4° C, and is used to treat hypoxemia is _____ .

1G. The substance that can exist as either a gas or liquid, is nonflammable but supports combustion, has a specific gravity of 1 (as a gas), and is made up of 78% nitrogen is _____ .

1H. _____ can be obtained as a by-product in the production of ammonia and lime and is purified by liquefaction and the fractional distillation process.

1I. Patients with severe airway obstruction may benefit from the use of what mixture of gases? _____ _____

1J. Which gas is used as a standard calibration gas for blood gas analyzers, certain transcutaneous monitors, and capnographs?

1K. Which gas can be produced by the physical separation of atmospheric air in patients' homes?

Think About This:
Why does inhaling helium make your voice sound strange?

2. Identify various types of medical gas cylinders (e.g., types 3, 3A, 3AA, and 3AL). (IIA9a)

2A. What three types of metal are used to construct seamless compressed-gas cylinders?

2B. What agency issues regulations for all cylinders used to store and transport compressed gases?

2C. Type 3 cylinders are made of _____ _____ .

2D. What type of cylinder is made from heat-treated, high-strength steel?

2E. What type of cylinder is constructed of specially prescribed seamless aluminum alloys?

2F. The filling pressure of a type 3AA "H" size cylinder is 2265 pound-force per square inch gauge (psig). What is the maximum amount of pressure this cylinder can hold?

Think About This:
Why are compressed-gas cylinders capable of holding 10% more than their maximum filling pressure?

3. Identify the following cylinder markings: Department of Transportation (DOT) specifications, service pressure, hydrostatic testing dates, manufacturer's identification, ownership mark, serial number, and cylinder size. (IIA9a)

Questions 3A through 3I refer to Figure 3-1.

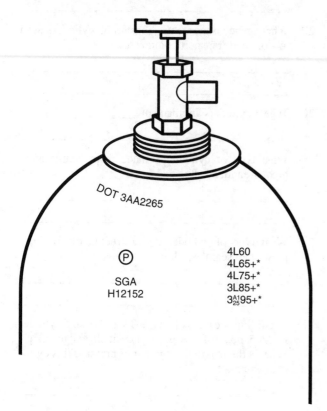

DOT 3AA2265

Ⓟ

SGA
H12152

4L60
4L65+*
4L75+*
3L85+*
3$_{25}^{A}$95+*

FIGURE 3-1

3A. From what type of metal is the cylinder in Figure 3-1 made?

_____

_____

3B. What is the service pressure for the cylinder in Figure 3-1?

_____

_____

3C. What year was the cylinder in Figure 3-1 last hydrostatically tested?

_____

_____

3D. What is the serial number for the cylinder in Figure 3-1?

_____

_____

3E. What is the manufacturer's mark on the cylinder in Figure 3-1?

_____

_____

3F. What is the year of the original hydrostatic test for the cylinder in Figure 3-1?

_____

_____

3G. What is the ownership mark on the cylinder in Figure 3-1?

_____

_____

3H. What size is the cylinder in Figure 3-1?

_____

_____

3I. Why should the cylinder in Figure 3-1 not be used at this time?

_____

_____

Think About This:

What should be done with a cylinder that has lost its elasticity?

4. List the color codes used to identify medical gas cylinders. (IIA9a)

	Gas	Color (in the United States)
4A.	Oxygen	
4B.	Nitrogen	
4C.	Helium	
4D.	Ethylene	
4E.	Cyclopropane	
4F.	Air	
4G.	Nitrous oxide	
4H.	Nitric oxide	
4I.	Helium/oxygen	
4J.	Carbon dioxide	
4K.	Carbon dioxide/oxygen	

4L. What are the two major exceptions to the international cylinder color-coding system?

_____

_____

Think About This:

Why are there two forms of identification for compressed-gas cylinders?

5. Discuss United States Pharmacopeia (USP) purity standards for medical gases. (IIA9a)

5A. What agency requires that compressed gases used for medical purposes meet certain minimum requirements for purity?

_____

_____

5B. Where is the purity of a gas indicated?

_____

_____

5C. Where are the purity standards for medical gases listed?

_____

_____

5D. Which gas has a purity standard of 97%?

_____

_____

5E. What is the purity standard for all medical gases except one?

_____

_____

Think About This:

Why are medical gases regulated for purity?

6. Compare the operation of direct-acting cylinder valves with diaphragm-type cylinder valves. (IIA9a)

Identify the common elements in Figure 3-2.

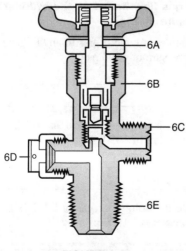

FIGURE 3-2

6A. _____

_____

6B. _____

_____

6C. _____

_____

6D. _____

_____

6E. _____

_____

Identify the common elements in Figure 3-3.

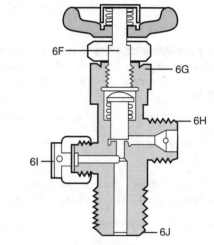

FIGURE 3-3

6F. _____

_____

6G. _____

_____

6H. _____

_____

6I. _____

_____

6J. _____

_____

6K. What is the difference between Figure 3-2 and Figure 3-3?

_____

_____

_____

_____

Chapter **3**   **Manufacture, Storage, and Transport of Medical Gases**

6L. Which type of cylinder valve can withstand pressures of more than 1500 psig?

_____

_____

6M. Which type of cylinder valve is preferred for use with flammable anesthetics? Why?

_____

_____

_____

_____

Think About This:

What type of valves should be used on cylinders used for *s*elf-contained *u*nderwater *b*reathing *a*pparatus (SCUBA) diving?

7. Explain the American Standards Association (ASA) indexing, the Pin Index Safety System (PISS), and the Diameter Index Safety System (DISS). (IIA9a)

7A. What is the purpose of cylinder safety systems?

_____

_____

7B. What safety system prevents an oxygen regulator from being placed on a large nitrous oxide cylinder?

_____

_____

7C. In which direction do non–life support gas cylinders thread?

_____

_____

7D. What safety system is used for small cylinders (size A to E)?

_____

_____

7E. How does the small-cylinder safety system differ from the large-cylinder safety system?

_____

_____

_____

_____

7F. Name the two safety systems that are used at station outlets.

_____

_____

Think About This:

With all the safety systems preventing the interchange of regulating equipment, is it still possible to hook up an oxygen-delivery device (i.e., a nasal cannula) to compressed air?

8. Identify and correct a problem with a cylinder valve assembly. (IIA9a)

8A. How would a respiratory therapist (RT) know whether there is a loose seal between a cylinder and a regulator?

_____

_____

_____

_____

8B. The RT prepares an "E" size cylinder for transport. When the RT turns the cylinder, there is a loud hissing noise. What is the most likely cause of the leak?

_____

_____

8C. What are two causes of low gas flow from a cylinder?

_____

_____

8D. Why should a cylinder valve not be opened up all the way?

_____

_____

_____

Think About This:

What would happen to an "H" size cylinder if the valve assembly were to be broken off?

9. Calculate the gas volume remaining in a compressed-gas cylinder, and estimate the duration of gas flow based on the cylinder's gauge pressure. (IIA9a)

9A. Calculate the volume of gas in an "E" size cylinder with a pressure of 1500 psig.

_____

_____

9B. Calculate the volume of gas in an "H" size cylinder with a pressure of 1050 psig.

_____

_____

9C. Calculate the volume of gas in a "G" size cylinder with a pressure of 1800 psig.

_____

_____

9D. Calculate the duration of gas flow for an "E" size cylinder with a pressure of 2200 psig and a flow of 3 L/min to a nasal cannula.

_____

_____

9E. Calculate the duration of gas flow for a "G" size cylinder with a pressure of 1600 psig and a flow of 6 L/min to an oxygen mask.

_____

_____

9F. Calculate the duration of gas flow, in hours, for an "H" size cylinder with a pressure of 1000 psig and a flow of 10 L/min to an oxygen device.

_____

_____

9G. An "H" size cylinder of oxygen contains 2000 psig of pressure, with a set flow of 12 L/min. How many hours will it take for this cylinder to get to 800 psig of pressure?

_____

_____

_____

_____

9H. A patient will be transferred from one hospital to another 50 miles away. The patient is receiving oxygen to his tracheostomy tube at a flow of 8 L/min. Travel time should be 1 hour. Will an "E" size cylinder with 1200 psig of pressure be able to last the trip? (*Support your answer with a mathematical calculation.*)

_____

_____

_____

_____

9I. A patient is being moved to the radiology department for a computed tomography scan. The round trip to radiology and the procedure will take 45 minutes. The patient is receiving oxygen via a nasal cannula at 2 L/min. The "E" size cylinder has 1000 psig of pressure. Is there enough gas in the cylinder for the procedure? (*Support your answer with a mathematical calculation.*)

_____

_____

_____

9J. Calculate how much time it will take for an "H" size cylinder with 800 psig of pressure to get to 200 psig of pressure with an oxygen device set at a flow rate of 4 L/min.

_____

_____

Think About This:
What other individuals need to calculate gas duration?

10. Describe the components of a bulk liquid oxygen system, and discuss National Fire Protection Association (NFPA) recommendations for the storage and use of liquid oxygen in bulk systems. (IIA9d)

Identify the components in Figure 3-4:

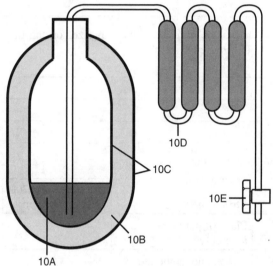

FIGURE 3-4

10A. _____

_____

10B. _____

_____

10C. _____

_____

10D. _____

_____

10E. _____

_____

10F. In Figure 3-4, where does the oxygen gas exist?

_____

_____

10G. Why are bulk liquid oxygen systems used in hospitals and large health care facilities?

_____

_____

_____

_____

10H. What is the NFPA definition of a *bulk oxygen system*?

_____

_____

_____

_____

_____

10I. What is the purpose of the vaporizer on the bulk liquid oxygen system?

_____

_____

_____

_____

Fill in the following table.

	Structure/Person	Distance from Bulk Oxygen System
10J.	Place of public assembly	
10K.	Nearest nonambulatory patient	
10L.	Public sidewalk	
10M.	Property line	
10N.	Parked vehicle	
10O.	Wood-frame structure	

Think About This:
Why shouldn't a child in a croup tent who is receiving oxygen play with a metal toy car?

11. Discuss the operation of a portable liquid oxygen system, and describe NFPA recommendations for these systems. (IIA9d)

11A. What are the main components of a home liquid oxygen system?

_____

_____

11B. The capacity of a stationary home unit is _____

_____, whereas the capacity

of a portable unit is _____

of liquid oxygen.

11C. What is the approximate working pressure of a portable liquid oxygen system?

_____

_____

11D. What is the purpose of the pressure-relief valve?

_____

_____

11E. How are portable liquid oxygen units filled?

_____

_____

11F. According to the NFPA, what actions should be taken if liquid oxygen comes in contact with the skin?

_____

_____

_____

_____

_____

_____

_____

_____

_____

Think About This:
Why does fog appear when a liquid oxygen spill occurs?

12. Calculate the duration of a portable liquid oxygen supply. (IIA9d)

12A. How long would a liquid oxygen supply weighing 8 lb last if a patient were receiving oxygen through a nasal cannula at 3 L/min?

_____

_____

_____

_____

12B. How long would a liquid oxygen supply weighing 12 lb last if a patient were receiving oxygen through a nasal cannula at 1.5 L/min?

_____

_____

_____

_____

12C. A portable liquid oxygen system weighs 1.5 lb when empty and 3.5 lb when full. How long will this system last when it is running at 1 L/min?

_____

_____

_____

_____

12D. How long will a portable liquid oxygen system containing 1.2 L of oxygen last when it is running at 2 L/min?

_____

_____

_____

_____

12E. Calculate the duration of a liquid oxygen supply if the liquid supply weighs 60 lb and is running at 3 L/min.

_____

_____

_____

_____

12F. Calculate the duration of a liquid oxygen supply when the empty container's weight is 6 lb, the full weight is 40 lb, and the oxygen flow is 5 L/min.

_____

_____

_____

_____

Think About This:

What use does the National Aeronautics and Space Administration (NASA) have for liquid oxygen?

13. Identify three types of medical air compressors, and describe the operational theory of each. (IIA9f)

Questions 13A through 13C refer to Figure 3-5.

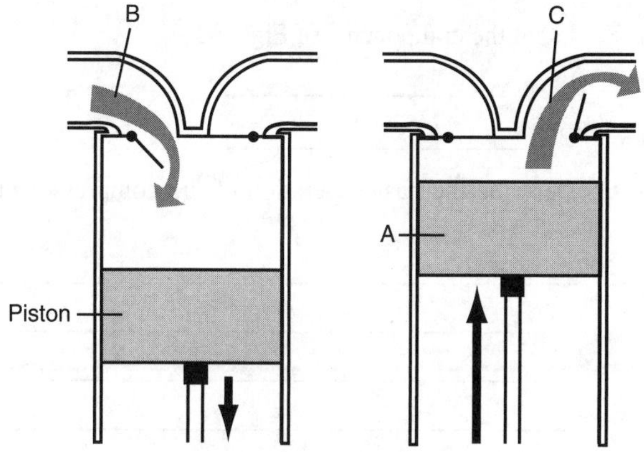

FIGURE 3-5

13A. What type of medical air compressor is shown in Figure 3-5?

_____

_____

13B. Label the components of Figure 3-5.

A. _____

B. _____

C. _____

13C. Describe the basic operation of the compressor in Figure 3-5.

_____

_____

_____

_____

_____

Questions 13D through 13F refer to Figure 3-6.

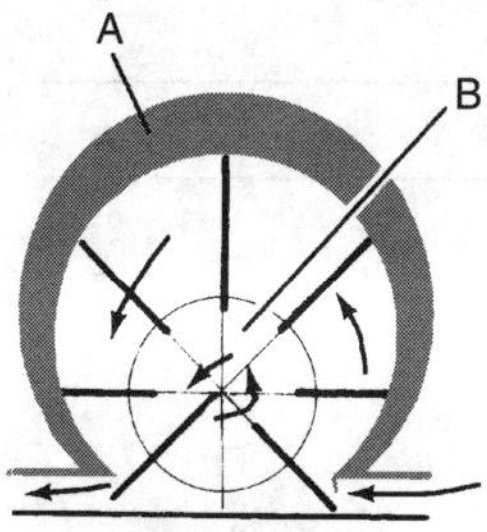

FIGURE 3-6

Chapter **3** **Manufacture, Storage, and Transport of Medical Gases**

13D. What type of medical air compressor is shown in Figure 3-6?

_____

_____

13E. Label the components of Figure 3-6.

A. _____

B. _____

13F. Describe the basic operation of the compressor in Figure 3-6.

_____

_____

_____

_____

_____

_____

Questions 13G through 13I refer to Figure 3-7.

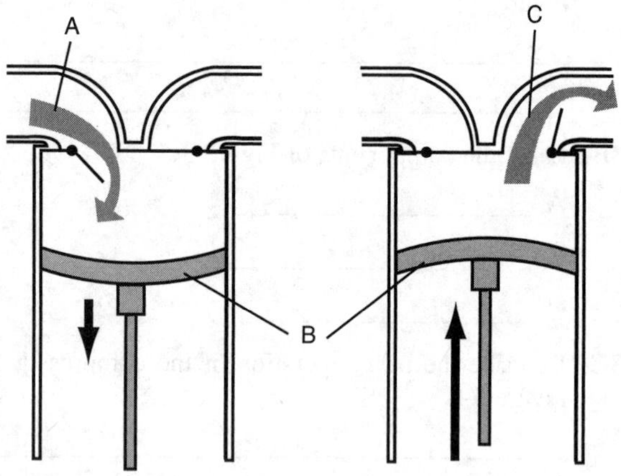

FIGURE 3-7

13G. What type of medical air compressor is shown in Figure 3-7?

_____

_____

13H. Label the components of Figure 3-7.

A. _____

B. _____

C. _____

13I. Describe the basic operation of the compressor in Figure 3-7.

_____

_____

_____

13J. Which type/types of compressors is/are best suited to provide 50 psig of pressure to mechanical ventilators?

_____

_____

Think About This:

What other applications do compressors have?

14. Summarize NFPA recommendations for medical air supply safety. (IIA9f)

14A. From what source must medical air come?

_____

_____

14B. What are the recommendations for where the air intake port should be located?

_____

_____

_____

_____

14C. What are the recommendations for the air taken into the system?

_____

_____

_____

14D. The minimum number of compressors recommended by the NFPA is _____.

14E. What dictates how many compressors a system should have?

_____

_____

14F. What determines the need for intake filters, after-coolers for air dryers, and additional downstream regulators?

_____

_____

14G. What features must air storage tanks or receivers have?

_____

_____

Think About This:

What are the everyday uses for compressed air?

15. Compare continuous supply systems with alternating central supply systems. (IIA9a)

15A. How many sources of gas supply does a continuous supply system have?

_____

_____

15B. What are the names for the gas sources in a continuous supply system?

_____

_____

15C. List four NFPA requirements for a continuous supply system.

_____

_____

_____

_____

15D. What would happen if the liquid source being used by a continuous supply system fails?

_____

_____

15E. Describe the gas sources for an alternating supply system.

_____

_____

_____

_____

_____

_____

15F. What happens when one of the gas sources in an alternating supply system becomes depleted?

_____

_____

_____

15G. When are switch signals activated in an alternating supply system?

_____

_____

15H. What type of central supply system is shown in Figure 3-8?

_____

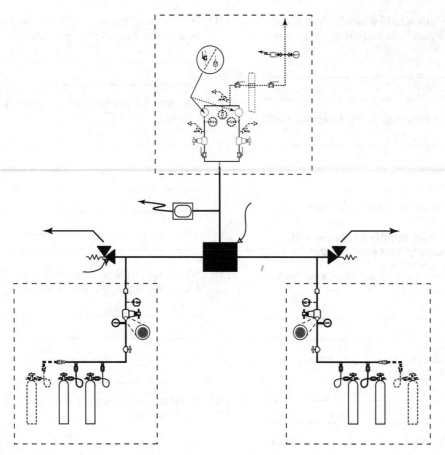

FIGURE 3-8
(From Kacmarek RM, Dimas S: *The essentials of respiratory care*, ed 4, St Louis, 2005, Mosby.)

Think About This:

What type of contingency plans should a hospital have for its central oxygen supply system during extreme weather?

16. Identify a DISS station outlet and a quick-connect station outlet. (IIA9a)

Questions 16A and 16B refer to Figure 3-9.

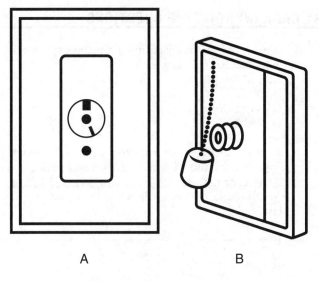

A   B

FIGURE 3-9

16A. Identify the type of station outlet in Figure 3-9*A*.

_____

_____

16B. Identify the type of station outlet in Figure 3-9*B*.

_____

_____

Think About This:

What would happen if all existing intensive care unit oxygen station outlets were purged with nitrogen?

17. Compare the operational theory of a membrane oxygenator with that of a molecular sieve oxygenator. (IIA9e)

17A. Describe the characteristics of the semipermeable membrane used in oxygen concentrators.

_____

_____

_____

_____

17B. How does a semipermeable membrane separate atmospheric gases?

_____

_____

_____

_____

17C. How does a semipermeable membrane oxygen concentrator provide a constant flow of atmospheric gas to the membrane?

_____

_____

17D. What is the usual output from an oxygen concentrator that uses a semipermeable membrane?

_____

_____

17E. How is nitrogen removed from the atmospheric gas in a molecular sieve oxygen concentrator?

_____

_____

17F. How many molecular sieves are contained in an oxygen concentrator?

_____

_____

17G. What is the pressure swing adsorption (PSA) method?

_____

_____

_____

17H. What is the typical output from a molecular sieve oxygen concentrator?

_____

_____

17I. The outlet pressure for a molecular sieve oxygen concentrator is _____

_____.

17J. Why can't regular oxygen flowmeters be used on molecular sieve oxygen concentrators?

_____

_____

_____

Think About This:

There are now portable oxygen concentrators that weigh less than 5 lb.

35

NATIONAL BOARD FOR RESPIRATORY CARE (NBRC)–TYPE QUESTIONS

1. An "E" size cylinder, with 1500 psig of pressure and set at a flow rate of 3 L/min will last how long?
   A. 0.2 hour
   B. 2.3 hours
   C. 20.1 hours
   D. 26.2 hours

2. The duration of oxygen flow for an "H" size cylinder with 2000 psig of pressure running at 6 L/min will be which of the following?
   A. 1.6 hours
   B. 11.9 hours
   C. 17.4 hours
   D. 23.7 hours

3. A full liquid oxygen cylinder weighs 10 lb; when empty, it weighs 2.5 lb. How many liters of oxygen does this liquid cylinder contain when it is full?
   A. 2 L
   B. 3 L
   C. 4 L
   D. 5 L

4. If the net weight of liquid oxygen in a cylinder is 3 lb, how long will the liquid oxygen last if the oxygen flow is running at 1.5 L/min?
   A. 4 hours 29 minutes
   B. 11 hours 28 minutes
   C. 28 hours 40 minutes
   D. 34 hours 24 minutes

5. An RT sets up an "E" size oxygen cylinder to transport a patient. When the cylinder is turned on, a loud whistling noise is heard from the cylinder. The most appropriate action is which of the following?
   A. Replace the regulator.
   B. Check the plastic washer.
   C. Loosen the regulator.
   D. Check for cross-threading.

6. Safety systems used at station outlets include which of the following?
   1. American Standards Safety System
   2. PISS
   3. DISS
   4. Quick-connect
   A. 1 and 3
   B. 1 and 2
   C. 2 and 4
   D. 3 and 4

7. What is the gaseous capacity of a liquid oxygen cylinder that has 0.52 L when full?
   A. 172 L
   B. 30 L
   C. 447 L
   D. 452 L

8. A stationary liquid oxygen system contains 80 lb of oxygen when full. A home care patient is using it 8 hours each day, during sleep, at a rate of 3 L/min. At this usage, how many days will the liquid oxygen last?
   A. 6
   B. 8
   C. 19
   D. 27

9. Which of the following "E" size oxygen cylinders will run out of oxygen first?

Cylinder	Pressure (in psig)	Flow (in L/min)
A.	700	0.5
B.	900	1.5
C.	1100	2
D.	1600	3

10. The liquid capacity of a full stationary liquid oxygen system is 35 L, and the home care patient is using it 7 hours per night with a flow rate of 1.5 L/min. Based on this usage, the number of days that this liquid oxygen system will last is which of the following?
    A. 14 days
    B. 33 days
    C. 41 days
    D. 47 days

Administering Medical Gases: Regulators, Flowmeters and Controlling Devices

4

Upon completion of this chapter, you will be able to:
1. Compare the design and operation of single-stage and multistage regulators.
2. Identify the components of preset and adjustable regulators.
3. Explain the operational theory of a Thorpe tube flowmeter, a Bourdon flowmeter, and a flow restrictor.
4. Demonstrate a method for determining whether or not a flowmeter is pressure-compensated.
5. Compare low-flow and high-flow oxygen-delivery systems.
6. Name several commonly used low-flow oxygen-delivery systems.
7. Discuss the advantages and disadvantages of oxygen-conserving devices.
8. Explain the operational theory of air-entrainment devices.
9. Compare the operation of oxygen blenders with that of oxygen mixers and adders.
10. Describe the physiologic effects of hyperbaric oxygen therapy.
11. List the indications and contraindications of nitric oxide therapy.
12. Describe the appropriate use of mixed-gas (e.g., heliox, carbogen) therapy.

"What oxygen is to the lungs, such is hope to the meaning of life."
Emil Brunner

Chapter **4 Administering Medical Gases: Regulators, Flowmeters and Controlling Devices**

ACHIEVING THE OBJECTIVES

1. Compare the design and operation of single-stage and multistage regulators. (IIA9a)

1A. What divides the body of a single-stage regulator in half?

_____

_____

1B. How is excessively high pressure handled by a single-stage regulator?

_____

_____

1C. What are the two opposing forces that dictate flow into the high-pressure side of the single-stage regulator?

_____

_____

1D. What closes the valve stem in a single-stage regulator?

_____

_____

_____

1E. How can a multistage regulator be easily identified?

_____

_____

1F. How is gas pressure reduced in a two-stage regulator?

_____

_____

_____

_____

_____

1G. The regulator that can control gas pressures with more precision is a _____.

1H. What is the difference between a single-stage regulator and a multistage regulator?

_____

_____

1I. The desired working pressure for respiratory therapy equipment is how many pounds per square inch (psi)?

_____

_____

1J. When incoming gas pressure is greater than the spring tension in the ambient chamber, what happens to the inlet valve?

_____

_____

Questions 1K and 1L refer to Figure 4-1.

1K. What type of regulator is shown in Figure 4-1?

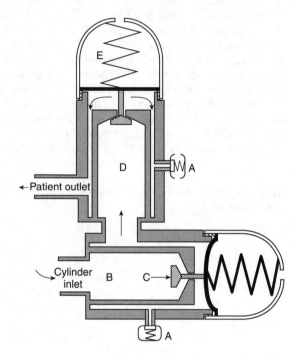

FIGURE 4-1

_____

_____

1L. Identify the components of Figure 4-1.

A. _____

B. _____

C. _____

D. _____

E. _____

Think About This:

What commercial use does a gas regulator have?

2. Identify the components of preset and adjustable regulators. (IIA9a)

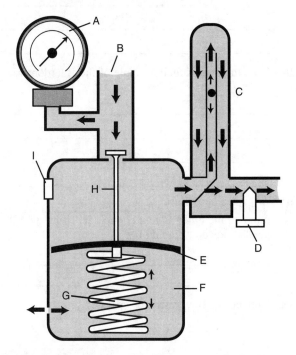

FIGURE 4-2
(Redrawn from Persing G: *Respiratory care exam review*, ed 3, St Louis, 2010, Saunders.)

In questions 2A through 2J, label the components identified with letters in Figure 4-2.

2A. "A"

_____

_____

2B. "B"

_____

_____

2C. "C"

_____

_____

2D. "D"

_____

_____

2E. "E"

_____

_____

2F. "F"

_____

_____

2G. "G"

_____

_____

2H. "H"

_____

_____

2I. "I"

_____

_____

2J. The type of regulator shown in Figure 4-2 is a

_____

_____.

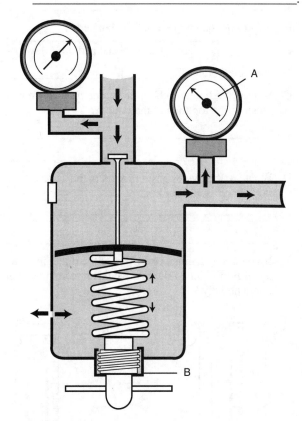

FIGURE 4-3
(Redrawn from Persing G: *Respiratory care exam review*, ed 3, St Louis, 2010, Saunders.)

In questions 2K and 2L, label the components identified with letters in Figure 4-3.

2K. "A" _____

_____

2L. "B" _____

_____

Chapter **4** **Administering Medical Gases: Regulators, Flowmeters and Controlling Devices**

2M. The type of regulator shown in Figure 4-3 is a _____

_____ .

Think About This:

What is the typical pressure setting for an outdoor propane cooking tank?

3. Explain the operational theory of a Thorpe tube flowmeter, a Bourdon flowmeter, and a flow restrictor. (IIA9a)

3A. Name the components of a Thorpe tube flowmeter.

_____

_____

_____

_____

3B. Adult flowmeters are usually calibrated in _____

_____ , whereas neonatal and pediatric flowmeters are calibrated in _____ .

3C. Why is the hollow tube of a Thorpe tube flowmeter wider at the top than at the bottom?

_____

_____

3D. What are the two opposing forces in the Thorpe tube flowmeter?

_____

_____

3E. If you put your finger over part of the outlet in flowmeter *B* in Figure 4-4, what would happen to the ball float and why?

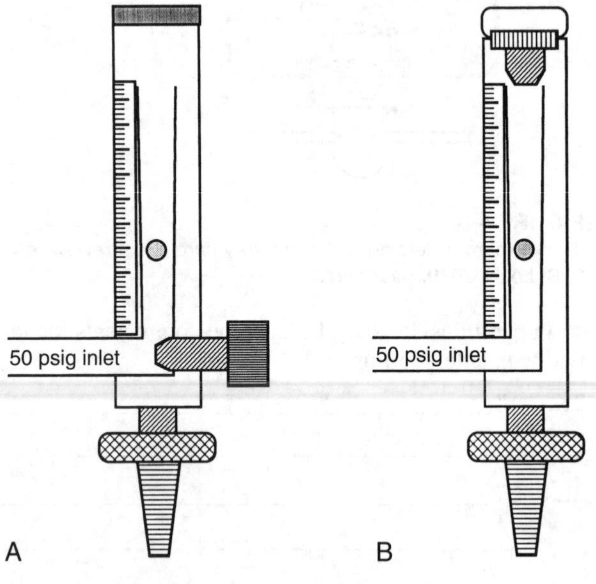

A   B

FIGURE 4-4

_____

_____

_____

_____

3F. State the operational principle of the Bourdon flowmeter.

_____

_____

_____

3G. If the flow from a Bourdon flowmeter is set to 8 L/min and the outlet is totally occluded, what will the needle indicator reading be?

_____

_____

3H. How does a flow restrictor operate?

_____

_____

_____

3I. Name the two types of flow restrictors.

_____

_____

3J. In the home care setting, where would flow restrictors be used most?

_____

_____

Think About This:

How can flow restrictors in your home save you money?

4. Demonstrate a method for determining whether or not a flowmeter is pressure-compensated. (IIA9a)

4A. Without plugging in the flowmeter, what are two ways you can determine whether or not it is pressure-compensated?

_____

_____

_____

_____

_____

_____

_____

4B. What test can be performed to determine whether or not a Thorpe tube flowmeter is pressure-compensated?

_____

_____

4C. Which of the two Thorpe tube flowmeters in Figure 4-4 is not back-pressure–compensated? Why?

_____

_____

_____

_____

Think About This:

Which type of Thorpe tube flowmeter would be most accurate to use in a hospital?

5. Compare low-flow and high-flow oxygen-delivery systems. (IIA1a)

5A. Why are low-flow devices also called *variable-performance devices*?

_____

_____

_____

_____

_____

5B. Name three factors that cause the fraction of inspired oxygen (F_IO_2) of a low-flow device to vary.

_____

_____

5C. Why are high-flow devices also called *fixed-performance devices*?

_____

_____

_____

_____

5D. How much can low-flow device F_IO_2 levels vary?

_____

_____

5E. What is the range for high-flow device F_IO_2 levels?

_____

_____

5F. A patient has been receiving supplemental oxygen via a low-flow device for 2 days. The patient's breathing becomes shallow. How would the F_IO_2 level when the patient is breathing with a normal tidal volume compare with the F_IO_2 level when the breathing is shallow? Why?

_____

_____

_____

_____

5G. A patient has been receiving supplemental oxygen via a high-flow device for 2 days. The patient's breathing becomes shallow. How would the F_IO_2 level when the patient is breathing with a normal tidal volume compare with the F_IO_2 level when the breathing is shallow? Why?

_____

_____

_____

_____

5H. When is a low-flow oxygen device appropriate for patient use?

_____

_____

5I. When is a high-flow oxygen device appropriate for patient use?

_____

_____

Think About This:

When can a high-flow oxygen device become a low-flow device?

6. Name several commonly used low-flow oxygen delivery systems. (IIA1a)

6A. Which low-flow oxygen-delivery device is most often used to treat hypoxemic patients who are breathing spontaneously?

_____

_____

Chapter **4** **Administering Medical Gases: Regulators, Flowmeters and Controlling Devices**

6B. Name three common problems related to the use of the device from question 6A.

_____

_____

_____

_____

6C. What is the theoretical oxygen concentration for use of the aforementioned low-flow oxygen device for adult patients? For pediatric patients?

_____

_____

_____

6D. What F_IO_2 level can a simple mask deliver?

_____

_____

6E. Why is 5 L/min the minimum flow for a simple mask?

_____

_____

6F. List at least four disadvantages of simple oxygen masks.

_____

_____

_____

_____

6G. What is the structural difference between a simple mask and a partial rebreathing mask?

_____

_____

6H. What happens to the patient's anatomic dead space volume during exhalation with a partial rebreathing mask in use?

_____

_____

6I. Why does the anatomic dead space of a patient using a partial rebreathing mask have a high F_IO_2 level?

_____

_____

_____

6J. What F_IO_2 range can a disposable partial rebreathing mask deliver?

_____

_____

6K. What is the structural difference between a partial rebreathing mask and a non-rebreathing mask?

_____

_____

_____

_____

6L. What F_IO_2 range can a disposable non-rebreathing mask deliver?

_____

6M. How is the appropriate oxygen flow rate determined for a reservoir-type mask?

_____

_____

_____

6N. Name the oxygen-conserving device that requires surgery for placement.

_____

_____

6O. Why can *transtracheal oxygen* (TTO) therapy make use of very low oxygen flow rates to achieve a desired level of oxygenation?

_____

_____

Think About This:

How can you change a non-rebreathing mask into a partial rebreathing mask?

7. Discuss the advantages and disadvantages of oxygen-conserving devices. (IIA9b)

Complete the following chart.

Oxygen-Conserving Device	Advantages	Disadvantages
7A.	7B.	7C.
7D.	7E.	7F.
7G.	7H.	7I.

Questions 7J and 7K refer to Figure 4-5.

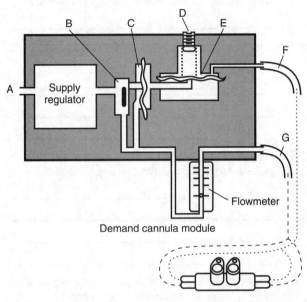

FIGURE 4-5
(Redrawn from Barnes TA: *Core textbook of respiratory care practice*, ed 2, St Louis, 1994, Mosby.)

7J. What is the inlet pressure (Figure 4-5*A*) for the demand cannula module?

_____

_____

7K. Label the letters *B* through *G* in Figure 4-5, the demand cannula module.

B. _____

_____

C. _____

_____

D. _____

_____

E. _____

_____

F. _____

_____

G. _____

_____

Think About This:

If you required home oxygen, which type of oxygen-conserving device would you want to have?

8. Explain the operational theory of air-entrainment devices. (IIA1b)

8A. What are the three factors that dictate the concentration of oxygen delivered by an air-entrainment device?

(1) _____

_____

(2) _____

_____

(3) _____

_____.

8B. How does the oxygen exiting the jet nozzle become diluted to a specific oxygen concentration?

_____

_____

_____

_____

8C. How do most commercially available air-entrainment masks vary oxygen concentration?

_____

_____

8D. What happens to the F_IO_2 when there is a partial obstruction of the gas flow downstream or partial obstruction of the entrainment ports?

_____

_____

_____

_____

Chapter **4** **Administering Medical Gases: Regulators, Flowmeters and Controlling Devices**

8E. Calculate the air-to-oxygen ratio, using Figure 4-6, when the F_IO_2 of an air-entrainment device is 45%.

```
        O₂              Air
       100              20
        ┌───────────────┐
        │ \           / │
        │   \       /   │
        │     \   /     │
        │   ──── %      │
        │     /   \     │
        │   /       \   │
        │ ↙           ↘ │
        └───────────────┘
      ┌───┐           ┌───┐
      └───┘           └───┘
   Ratio   1            ___
```

FIGURE 4-6

_____

8F. What are the total parts for 45%?

_____

_____

8G. Calculate the total flow for a 45% air-entrainment device when the oxygen flow is set to 10 L/min.

_____

_____

8H. What happens to the actual delivered F_IO_2 when a patient's inspiratory demand exceeds the total flow of an air-entrainment device?

_____

_____

_____

_____

8I. At what F_IO_2 range do air-entrainment masks function appropriately?

_____

_____

8J. Calculate the total flow for a 35% air-entrainment mask with a set oxygen flow rate of 8 L/min.

_____

_____

8K. Accumulated moisture in the tubing of an air-entrainment large-volume nebulizer will cause what to happen to the delivered F_IO_2?

_____

_____

Think About This:

What are some practical uses of the Venturi effect?

9. Compare the operation of oxygen blenders with that of oxygen mixers and adders. (IIA9a)

9A. What are the components of a typical oxygen-adder system?

_____

_____

9B. With an oxygen-adder system, how can an F_IO_2 of 35% be achieved?

_____

_____

_____

_____

9C. What are the components of an oxygen blender?

_____

_____

_____

_____

_____

_____

9D. Why does an oxygen blender require a filter for the gases entering the blender housing?

_____

_____

_____

9E. What device is most reliable for providing a variety of F_IO_2 levels for mechanical ventilators?

_____

_____

Think About This:

What are the similarities and differences between an oxygen blender and the blender you use to make food or drinks?

10. Describe the physiologic effects of hyperbaric oxygen therapy.

10A. What are the two problems that hyperbaric therapy was originally used to treat?

_____

_____

10B. List six other disorders that hyperbaric therapy is used to treat.

_____

_____

_____

10C. What happens to lung volumes during hyperbaric therapy?

_____

_____

_____

10D. Which gas law explains what happens to the alveolar and arterial partial pressures of oxygen (P_AO_2 and $PaCO_2$ respectively) during hyperbaric therapy?

_____

_____

10E. Calculate the P_AO_2 during hyperbaric therapy when the barometric pressure (P_{bar}) equals 3 atm, F_IO_2 equals 1, $PaCO_2$ equals 45 mm Hg, and water vapor pressure is 47 mm Hg.

_____

_____

_____

10F. Which gas law explains the changes in the PaO_2 that occur with exposure to hyperbaric therapy?

_____

_____

10G. Calculate the oxygen-carrying capacity of plasma when P_{bar} equals 3 atm, F_IO_2 equals 1, $PaCO_2$ equals 45 mm Hg, and water vapor pressure is 47 mm Hg.

_____

_____

_____

_____

10H. Calculate the oxygen-carrying capacity of plasma when P_{bar} equals 2.5 atm, F_IO_2 equals 1, $PaCO_2$ equals 40 mm Hg, and water vapor pressure is 47 mm Hg.

_____

_____

10I. What gas law would cause the temperature within a hyperbaric chamber to rise when pressure is exerted?

_____

_____

10J. How is temperature controlled within a hyperbaric chamber?

_____

_____

10K. Why is hyperbaric oxygen therapy useful in the treatment of skin grafts?

_____

_____

10L. Why is hyperbaric oxygen therapy used to treat anaerobic infections?

_____

_____

_____

_____

Think About This:

What neurologic disorders may be treated with hyperbaric oxygen therapy?

11. List the indications and contraindications for nitric oxide therapy. (IIA26)

11A. What property does nitric oxide have that makes it useful in the treatment of various pulmonary disorders?

_____

11B. List the indications for nitric oxide therapy.

_____

_____

_____

_____

11C. How is nitric oxide supplied?

_____

_____

11D. The by-products of nitric oxide and oxygen and water are:

_____ and _____

_____.

11E. The therapeutic dose of nitric oxide is between ___

_____ and

_____.

11F. What three gases are monitored during nitric oxide therapy?

_____

_____

Think About This:

What physiologic and cellular processes does nitric oxide play a role in within the body?

45

12. Describe the appropriate use of mixed-gas (e.g., heliox, carbogen) therapy. (IIA15)

12A. How are heliox mixtures supplied?

_____

_____

12B. What property of heliox makes it useful in the treatment of certain respiratory problems?

_____

_____

12C. List five indications for heliox therapy.

(1) _____

_____

(2) _____

_____

(3) _____

_____

(4) _____

_____

(5) _____

_____

12D. Calculate the actual flow for an 80:20 heliox mixture being delivered to a patient via an oxygen flowmeter set at 10 L/min.

_____

_____

12E. The reservoir bag of a non-rebreathing mask needs to be maintained at 12 L/min to keep from collapsing. A 70:30 mixture of heliox is now connected to this mask. Calculate the set flow needed for actual heliox mixture to be 12 L/min.

_____

_____

_____

_____

12F. Calculate the actual flow for a 60:40 heliox mixture being delivered to a patient via an oxygen flowmeter set at 8 L/min.

_____

_____

12G. An insufficient amount of oxygen in the heliox mixture can result in:

_____

_____

12H. List four indications for carbogen.

(1) _____

(2) _____

(3) _____

(4) _____

12I. What are the clinical manifestations of carbon dioxide toxicity?

_____

_____

_____

12J. How is carbogen supplied?

_____

_____

12K. What mask should be used to deliver carbogen?

_____

_____

12L. During carbogen therapy, what should the respiratory therapist (RT) be monitoring to help prevent carbon dioxide toxicity?

_____

_____

_____

_____

Think About This:

How should a small-volume nebulizer be set up to deliver aerosolized medication with heliox?

NATIONAL BOARD FOR RESPIRATORY CARE (NBRC)–TYPE QUESTIONS

1. Spring tension and gas pressure are the two opposing forces in which of the following?
   A. Bourdon gauge
   B. Kinetic tube
   C. Flowmeter
   D. Regulator

2. When a closed Thorpe tube flowmeter is attached to a 50-psi oxygen source, the indicator float jumps up, then quickly falls to 0. This flowmeter is which of the following?
   A. Broken
   B. A Bourdon gauge flowmeter
   C. Compensated for back pressure
   D. Uncompensated for back pressure

3. Absorption atelectasis and oxygen toxicity may occur with which of the following?
   A. $F_IO_2 < 0.30$
   B. $F_IO_2 < 0.70$
   C. $F_IO_2 \geq 0.50$
   D. $F_IO_2 = 0.50$

4. A patient is receiving oxygen via a nasal cannula at 3 L/min. The patient's respiratory rate and tidal volume have decreased significantly. The F_IO_2 will do which of the following?
   A. Increase
   B. Stabilize
   C. Decrease
   D. Not change

5. A home care patient calls to inform the RT that his transtracheal catheter (TTC) accidentally fell out last night and that he was unable to reinsert it. The RT should tell the patient to do which of the following?
   A. Insert a dilating or stenting device.
   B. Continue attempts to reinsert the catheter.
   C. Use a nasal cannula and call his physician as soon as possible.
   D. Use a nasal cannula until another TTC is delivered to the home.

6. How much air will be entrained when a person is using a 35% air-entrainment adapter with 8 L/min oxygen?
   A. 35 L/min
   B. 40 L/min
   C. 45 L/min
   D. 55 L/min

7. If 35 L/min of humidified oxygen is added to 10 L/min of humidified air, what is the resultant F_IO_2?
   A. 0.82
   B. 0.74
   C. 0.40
   D. 0.38

8. A patient requires 15 L/min to prevent the reservoir bag on a non-rebreathing mask from collapsing. For an 80:20 heliox mixture, what is the correct flow rate to maintain the reservoir bag?
   A. 8 L/min
   B. 15 L/min
   C. 24 L/min
   D. 27 L/min

9. Which type of oxygen-delivery device should be used in the treatment of smoke inhalation?
   A. Nasal cannula at 6 L/min
   B. Simple mask at 10 L/min
   C. Non-rebreathing mask at 15 L/min
   D. Large-volume aerosol nebulizer at 0.6 setting

10. A home care patient reports no oxygen coming out of his pulse demand oxygen system. What are the probable causes?
    1. Flow set too low
    2. Improperly placed sensor
    3. Decreased power or no power to the unit
    4. Solenoid valve not properly opening
       A. 1 and 4 only
       B. 1 and 2 only
       C. 2 and 3 only
       D. 2 and 4 only

11. The work of breathing of a patient with limited lung reserves will increase with increased ambient pressure because of which of the following?
    A. Increased gas density
    B. Decreased gas volume
    C. Increased gas temperature
    D. Decreased oxygen solubility

Chapter **4** **Administering Medical Gases: Regulators, Flowmeters and Controlling Devices**

Airway Management Devices and Advanced Cardiac Life Support

LEARNING OBJECTIVES

Upon completion of this chapter, you will be able to:
1. Recognize normal airway anatomy.
2. Describe a complete airway exam.
3. Describe ways to displace the tongue to improve gas exchange in unconscious patients.
4. List patient characteristics that may contribute to a difficult mask ventilation or intubation.
5. List several complications resulting from improper placement of oral and nasopharyngeal airways.
6. Explain how to place the laryngeal mask airway (LMA) and the Combitube in unconscious patients.
7. Describe the appropriate sequence of steps for inserting an endotracheal tube (ETT) using laryngoscopy in order to provide a secure airway.
8. Identify three ways to confirm proper placement of an ETT.
9. Name three airway devices that can facilitate the placement of an ETT in the event of a difficult laryngoscopy.
10. Identify the airway risks facing intubated patients and identify strategies to avoid, and equipment used to treat, these complications.
11. Identify the equipment necessary to perform invasive ventilation (transtracheal or surgical airway), and describe a procedure for airway entry.
12. Review the equipment and steps used to obtain sputum samples from patients with endotracheal and tracheostomy tubes.
13. Describe three ways to wean patients from tracheostomy tubes (TTs).
14. List three methods that allow patients with TTs to speak.
15. Identify various types of manual resuscitators, and discuss the common hazards associated with the use of these devices.
16. Understand changes in advanced cardiac life support (ACLS) regarding the prioritization of airway management and chest compressions.

"There is a single light of science, and to brighten it anywhere is to brighten it everywhere."
Isaac Asimov

ACHIEVING THE OBJECTIVES

1. Recognize normal airway anatomy.

1A. Label the parts of Figure 5-1.

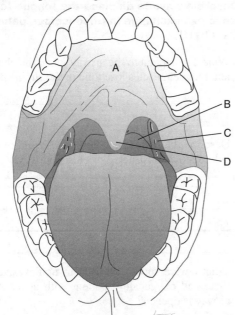

FIGURE 5-1

A. _____ hard palate _____
B. _____ oropharynx _____
C. _____ tonsils _____
D. _____ uvula _____

1B. Label the parts of Figure 5-2.

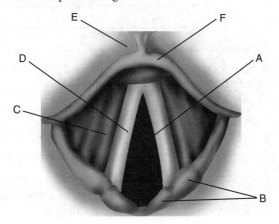

FIGURE 5-2

A. _____
B. _____
C. _____
D. _____

E. _____
F. _____

1C. The narrowest portion of an adult's airway is

_____.

1D. The narrowest portion of a child's airway until age 6 is the

_____.

1E. Match the following upper airway anatomy with its nerve innervations.

Anatomic Structure	Nerve
___(1) Anterior portion of the tongue	(a) Recurrent laryngeal nerves (CN X)
___(2) Posterior third of the tongue	(b) External branch of superior laryngeal nerve (CN X)
___(3) Vocal cords	(c) Internal branch of superior laryngeal nerve (CN X)
___(4) Underside of the epiglottis	(d) Trigeminal nerve (CN V)
___(5) Trachea below the vocal cords	(e) Glossopharyngeal nerve (CN IX)
___(6) Muscles of larynx	(f) Superior laryngeal nerve
___(7) Cricothyroid muscles	(g) Vagus nerve

Think About This:

How do the vocal cords produce sound?

2. Describe a complete airway examination. (IB1b)

2A. Why is an airway examination important?

_____

_____

2B. List five important points that may be obtained from an airway history, either from the patient or from review of the past medical records.

_____

_____

_____

_____

_____

2C. Name the common components of an airway examination.

_____

_____

_____

2D. The thyromental distance that is of concern when assessing the airway is

_____

_____

_____.

2E. What type of external neck anatomy is of concern with respect to a difficult airway?

_____

_____

2F. List indicators in the dentition that suggest intubation might be difficult.

_____

_____

_____

_____

2G. The Mallampati class for the airway shown in Figure 5-3 is _____.

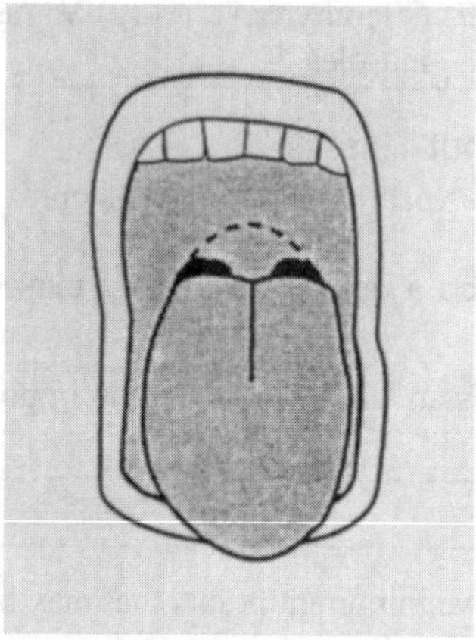

FIGURE 5-3

2H. List six predictors of a difficult intubation.

_____

_____

_____

_____

_____

_____

Think About This:
Should a person with a "difficult" airway wear a medical alert bracelet with that information?

3. Describe ways to displace the tongue to improve gas exchange in unconscious patients. (IIA7a, IIIG1f)

3A. What can happen to the airway when the pharyngeal and tongue muscles lose tone in the supine position?

_____

_____

3B. Describe the patient position that should be used to help open an obstructed or closed airway.

_____

_____

_____

_____

3C. What device should be used to noninvasively ventilate and oxygenate a patient with apnea after the airway is opened?

_____

_____

3D. How should this device (from question 3C) be applied when used on the patient?

_____

_____

_____

_____

_____

_____

3E. List four techniques that can be used to facilitate successful ventilation of a patient with apnea.

_____

_____

_____

_____

3F. Name and describe the two types of oropharyngeal airways available to displace the tongue.

_____

_____

_____

_____

3G. Describe three ways that an oropharyngeal airway may be placed in an unconscious person.

_____

_____

_____

_____

_____

_____

_____

_____

_____

Think About This:

What causes snoring?

4. List characteristics of the patient that may contribute to a difficult mask ventilation or intubation. (IIIG1f)

4A. The body mass index (BMI) that decreases the success of face mask ventilation (FMV) is a BMI of

_____

_____ .

4B. Which Mallampati airway classes are associated with an increased risk of difficulty in providing FMV?

_____

_____

4C. The age at which increased difficulty in providing FMV may begin is

_____

_____ .

4D. The type of chin structure that is associated with increased difficulty in FMV is

_____

_____ .

4E. Name three additional factors that are associated with increased difficulty in FMV.

_____

_____

4F. The only easily modifiable risk factor for poor FMV is the presence of

_____

_____ .

Think About This:

Why should face masks accompany all intubated patients during transport?

5. List several complications resulting from improper placement of oral and nasopharyngeal airways. (IIA7a)

5A. What is the consequence of the use of a Guedel or Berman airway that is one size too small?

_____

_____

5B. What will happen if oropharyngeal airway placement is attempted on a patient with intact airway protective reflexes?

_____

_____

5C. If a patient forcibly bites an oropharyngeal airway, what may happen?

_____

_____

5D. What complication is caused by a nasopharyngeal airway that is too long for a patient?

_____

_____

5E. A major complication of inserting a nasopharyngeal tube is _____ .

5F. What is the long-term risk of nasopharyngeal tube placement?

_____

_____

Think About This:

Should a nasotracheal airway be used in a patient with cranial trauma?

6. Explain how to place the laryngeal mask airway (LMA) and the Combitube in unconscious patients. (IIA7f, IIA7g, IIIB4a, IIIB4b)

6A. How does an LMA provide an airway for manual ventilation?

_____

_____

6B. List five reasons why the LMA is a useful emergency airway device.

_____

_____

_____

_____

6C. How should an LMA be checked for leaks?

_____

_____

6D. Describe how an LMA is inserted.

_____

_____

_____

_____

_____

_____

6E. The three methods used to check for correct placement of an LMA are:

_____

_____

_____

_____

_____.

6F. What size of LMA should be used for an 85-kg male patient?

_____

_____

6G. When is it appropriate to use a Combitube?

_____

_____

6H. What type of artificial airway would be most beneficial to use with a bloodied airway?

_____

_____

_____

6I. How is a Combitube inserted?

_____

_____

_____

_____

6J. Label the parts of the Combitube in Figure 5-4.

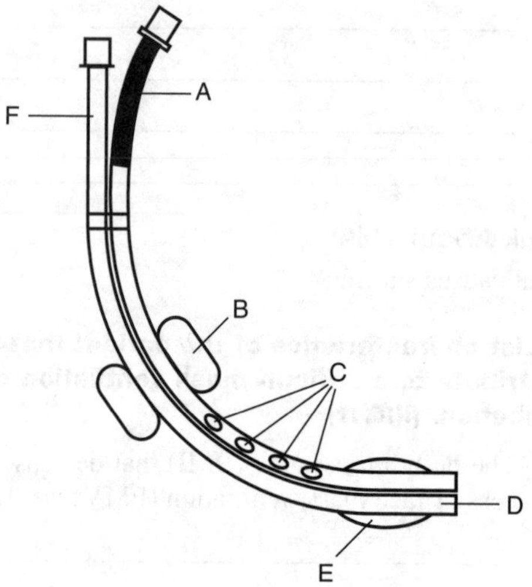

FIGURE 5-4

A. _____

B. _____

C. _____

D. _____

E. _____

F. _____

Think About This:

Why are there so many different types of artificial airways?

7. Describe the appropriate sequence of steps for inserting an endotracheal tube (ETT) using laryngoscopy in order to provide a secure airway. (IIA7b, IIA7e, IIIB3)

7A. What needs to be done for an apneic patient before intubation?

_____

_____

7B. Label the parts of the ETT in Figure 5-5.

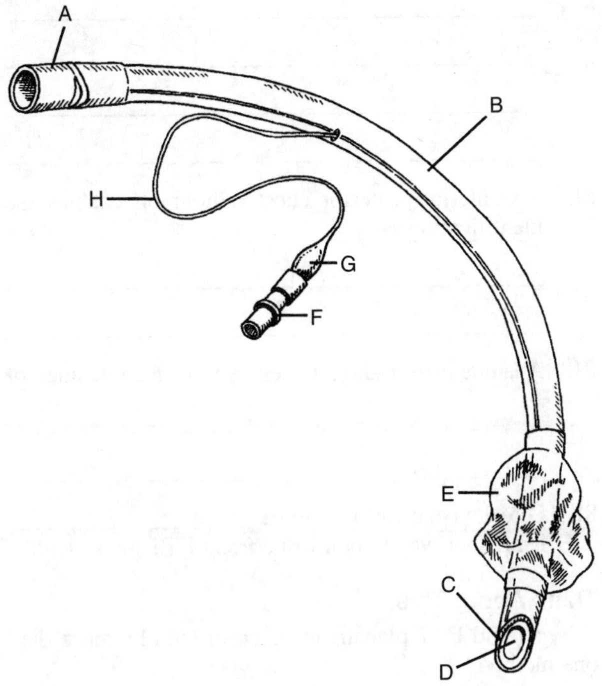

FIGURE 5-5
(From Sills JR: *The comprehensive respiratory therapist exam review*, ed 5, St Louis, 2010, Mosby.)

A. _____

B. _____

C. _____

D. _____

E. _____

F. _____

G. _____

H. _____

7C. Name and describe the two types of laryngoscope blades.

_____

_____

7D. How should a laryngoscope be held?

_____

_____

_____

7E. What is the correct placement for each of the two types of laryngoscope blades?

_____

_____

_____

_____

_____

_____

7F. Once in the appropriate place, how should the laryngoscope be moved to bring the epiglottis into view?

_____

_____

7G. List the equipment needed for endotracheal intubation.

_____

_____

_____

_____

_____

_____

_____

_____

7H. What size of laryngoscope blade should be used for an average adult? _____

7I. Place the sequence of events for intubation in the order that they should occur.

____Pass the ETT through the vocal cords.
____Check the placement of the ETT.
____Check laryngoscope, and check ETT cuff.
____Place lubricated stylet into the ETT.
____Lubricate the ETT with water-soluble lubricant.
____Inflate the cuff.
____Visualize the laryngeal structures with the laryngoscope.

7J. Why should cuff pressure be kept below 25 cm H_2O?

_____

_____

_____

Chapter **5** **Airway Management Devices and Advanced Cardiac Life Support**

Think About This:

How many intubations should a respiratory therapist (RT) perform in the operating room to become certified by her hospital?

8. Identify three ways to confirm proper placement of an ETT. (IB4a, IB7b, IC10, IIIB5)

8A. Why is confirmation of ETT placement important?

_____

_____

8B. What is the most sensitive method to confirm ETT placement?

_____

_____

8C. How does a color-change capnometer work?

_____

_____

8D. After intubation, a color-change capnometer is attached to the ETT, but it does not indicate a change in color. Give two reasons why this would happen.

_____

_____

_____

8E. How does the esophageal detection device work?

_____

_____

_____

8F. With what types of patients have false-positive and false-negative results been reported when esophageal detection devices are used?

_____

8G. Auscultation after intubation should be done in how many areas?

_____

_____

8H. Why can chest auscultation be misleading?

_____

_____

_____

8I. An anterior-posterior chest radiograph enables the identification of

_____

_____.

8J. A lateral chest radiograph enables the identification of

_____

_____.

8K. Direct visualization with a _____ is another way to confirm correct ETT placement.

Think About This:

Why should ETT placement be confirmed by more than one method?

9. Name three airway devices that can aid in placing an ETT in the event of a difficult laryngoscopy. (IIA7e)

9A. How is a *lightwand* or lighted stylet used to facilitate intubation of a difficult airway?

_____

_____

_____

_____

_____

_____

9B. List the situations when the use of a *lightwand* or lighted stylet is appropriate.

_____

_____

_____

_____

9C. The type of device that relies on lenses, mirrors, or fiberoptic technology to obtain a clear view of the glottic opening and cords is known as _____ _____.

9D. What is the "gold standard" for a known difficult airway or an unstable neck?

_____

_____

9E. Describe how the retrograde intubation technique is performed.

_____

_____

_____

_____

_____

_____

_____

_____

9F. Complete the following table.

Alternative Airway Device	Complications
Lighted stylet	
Laryngoscope, indirectly applied	
Flexible fiberoptic bronchoscope	
Retrograde wire	

Think About This:

Why is airway management the most important initial element in trauma management?

10. Identify the airway risks facing intubated patients and identify strategies to avoid, and equipment used to treat, these complications. (IIA7b, IIIB4c, IIIB8, IIIF2g1, IIIF2g2, IIIF2g3, IIIF2g4)

10A. An increase in mucus production or thickness can do what to an ETT?

_____

_____

10B. What is incorporated into the tip of ETTs that will decrease the likelihood of an ETT becoming occluded?

_____

_____

_____

_____

_____

10C. What will happen to the airway of a patient with an ETT that bent in half?

_____

_____

10D. Where do plastic ETTs tend to collapse?

_____

_____

10E. What type of equipment may be used to prevent a bend or kink in the ETT?

_____

_____

10F. Why are patients with ETTs at risk for dried secretions?

_____

_____

10G. What equipment should be used with intubated patients to prevent the drying of secretions?

_____

_____

10H. What other normal physiologic function is compromised because of the presence of an ETT?

_____

_____

10I. How can secretions be mobilized in a patient who has an endotracheal or tracheostomy tube?

_____

_____

10J. How can inadvertent movement or extubation of ETTs be prevented?

_____

_____

_____

_____

10K. What will happen to the airway if the ETT cuff fails to hold pressure?

_____

_____

10L. The most appropriate action to take when there is a cuff failure is to _____

_____ by using a/an _____

_____.

10M. What happens to the integrity of the airway when there is a leak in the pilot balloon?

_____

_____

10N. What equipment and method may be used to overcome a leaky pilot balloon?

_____

_____

_____

_____

Think About This:

How is an artificial airway secured on a giraffe?

11. Identify the equipment necessary to perform invasive ventilation (i.e., a transtracheal or surgical airway), and describe a procedure for airway entry. (III.I3d)

11A. In case of an unsuccessful intubation attempt, where a patent airway has not been established and manual ventilation is not possible, what method should be used to establish an emergency airway?

_____

_____

11B. Where, on Figure 5-6, should this emergency airway be located?

_____

_____

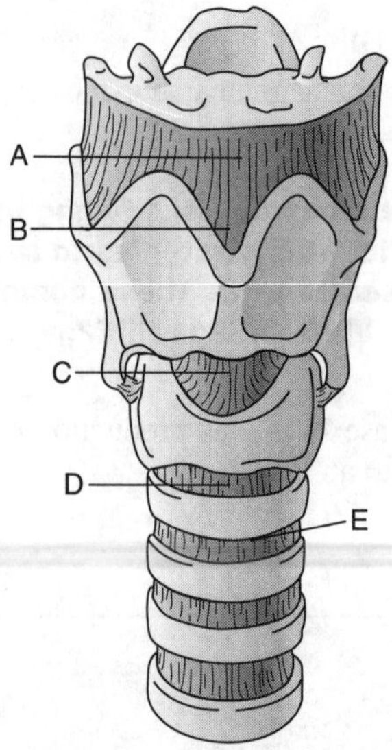

FIGURE 5-6
(From Kacmarek RM, Dimas S: *The essentials of respiratory care*, ed 4, St Louis, 2005, Mosby.)

11C. List the equipment necessary to establish this emergency airway.

_____

_____

_____

_____

11D. Describe the procedure for establishing this emergency airway.

_____

_____

_____

_____

_____

_____

_____

_____

_____

_____

11E. Identify the location for a percutaneous dilatory tracheostomy (PDT) on Figure 5-6.

_____

11F. List the equipment necessary for the Ciaglia PDT method.

_____

_____

11G. What equipment may be used to help prevent inadvertent injury of the membranous posterior tracheal wall?

_____

_____

11H. What is the main difference between the Ciaglia PDT method and the tracheostomy method described by Griggs?

_____

_____

_____

_____

11I. A single, tapered dilator that is used instead of sequential dilators is known as the _____

_____.

Think About This:

Can nonhuman animals live with tracheotomies?

12. Review the equipment and steps used to obtain sputum samples from patients with endotracheal and tracheostomy tubes. (IIA8, IIA21, IIB5, IIIC2, IIID9, IIIF2h)

12A. What physiologic functions are bypassed with invasive artificial airways?

_____

_____

_____

_____

12B. What vacuum pressures must the vacuum system be able to generate?

_____

_____

12C. What personal protective equipment should be available for suctioning patients by using invasive artificial airways?

_____

_____

12D. The RT should be continually observing what three factors during the suctioning process?

_____

_____

12E. To prevent hypoxemia during the suctioning, what should be done before beginning the process?

_____

_____

12F. How far down into the trachea should the catheter be placed?

_____

_____

12G. When should suctioning be applied?

_____

_____

12H. Suction should be applied for how long in the trachea?

_____

_____

12I. Place the sequence of events in order for suctioning the airway of a patient by using an invasive artificial airway.

___Preoxygenate with 100% oxygen for 30 to 60 seconds.
___Don personal protective wear.
___Repeat the procedure as needed.
___Check equipment.
___Gently withdraw the catheter with suction.
___Suction the patient's mouth and nose.
___Explain procedure to the patient.
___Allow the patient to rest.
___Attach the catheter to the vacuum system by using the aseptic technique.
___Advance catheter without suctioning until obstruction is detected.
___Note baseline heart rate, electrocardiographic rhythm, and pulse oximeter saturation.
___Wash hands.

12J. A size 7.5 (inner diameter) TT requires what size of suction catheter?

_____

Think About This:

What should you do if the electrocardiogram shows premature ventricular contractions during suctioning?

13. Describe three ways to wean patients from tracheostomy tubes (TTs). (IIA7c, IIID7)

13A. Describe the fastest way for a tracheostomy patient to be weaned from the TT.

_____

_____

13B. In what situation should a stoma be maintained?

_____

_____

13C. What type of TT can be used to maintain tracheal access while the patient is being "weaned" from the larger TT?

_____

_____

13D. What other device is available to maintain a tracheostomy stoma?

_____

_____

13E. Which device used to maintain a tracheostomy stoma has more advantages?

_____

_____

Think About This:

How do patients with permanent tracheostomies humidify inspired air?

14. List three methods that allow patients with TTs to speak. (IIA7d)

Questions 14A through 14C refer to Figure 5-7.

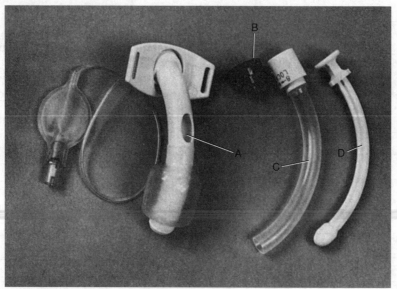

FIGURE 5-7
(From Kacmarek RM, Stoller JK, Heuer AJ: *Egan's fundamentals of respiratory care*, ed 10, St Louis, 2013, Mosby.)

14A. What type of TT is shown in Figure 5-7?

_____

_____

14B. Label the following parts of Figure 5-7.

A. _____

B. _____

C. _____

D. _____

14C. Explain how the TT in Figure 5-7 is used to allow speech.

_____

_____

_____

_____

_____

_____

14D. Name two other devices available to allow patients with TTs, who are capable of initiating and maintaining spontaneous ventilation, to speak.

_____

_____

14E. List two ways to create an open upper airway with a TT.

_____

_____

14F. What device is designed to allow speech in patients who are unable to sustain unaided ventilation?

_____

_____

14G. How does the device mentioned in 14F function?

_____

_____

_____

14H. What are the benefits of restoring the ability to speak to a patient with a TT?

_____

_____

_____

_____

Think About This:

Can patients with ETTs speak during ventilation?

15. Describe various types of manual resuscitators, and discuss the common hazards associated with the use of these devices. (IIA5)

15A. What is the function of a manual resuscitator?

_____

_____

15B. How are manual resuscitators classified?

_____

Questions 15C through 15F refer to Figure 5-8.

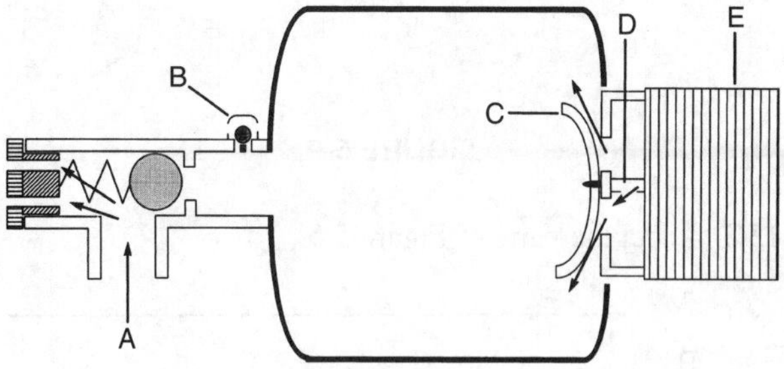

FIGURE 5-8

15C. Label the parts of Figure 5-8.

A. _____

B. _____

C. _____

D. _____

E. _____

15D. What type of manual resuscitator is shown in Figure 5-8? _____

15E. Which phase of ventilation is shown in Figure 5-8?

_____

15F. Describe how the manual resuscitator in Figure 5-8 works.

_____

_____

_____

_____

_____

_____

_____

_____

Questions 15G through 15J refer to Figure 5-9.

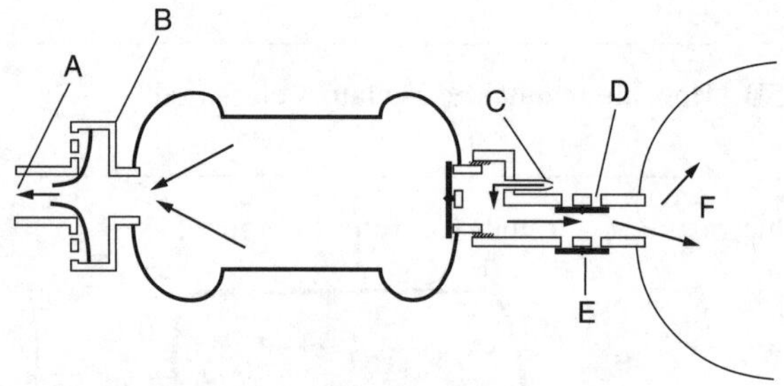

FIGURE 5-9

15G. Label the parts of Figure 5-9.

A. _____

B. _____

C. _____

D. _____

E. _____

15H. What type of manual resuscitator is shown in Figure 5-9? _____

_____

15I. Which phase of ventilation is shown in Figure 5-9?

_____

15J. Describe how the manual resuscitator in Figure 5-9 works.

_____

_____

_____

_____

_____

_____

_____

15K. The American Hospital Association specifies that a manual resuscitator should deliver a tidal volume of _____ to a patient.

15L. List three causes of hypoventilation during manual ventilation.

_____

_____

_____

15M. When would high airway pressures most likely be encountered during manual ventilation?

_____

_____

15N. Excessively high pressures during manual ventilation increase the patient's risk of developing what?

_____

_____ .

Think About This:

Should manual resuscitators be kept with every automated external defibrillator?

16. Understand changes in advanced cardiac life support (ACLS) regarding the prioritization of airway management and chest compressions. (III.I.1.b)

16A. The 2010 guidelines from the American Heart Association (AHA) no longer recommends _____ during bystander CPR.

16B. Identify the primary goal for CPR under the 2010 AHA guidelines.

_____

_____

16C. Identify the primary two reasons for the revised guidelines.

_____

_____

Think About This:

How do the 2010 AHA guidelines apply to health care providers?

NATIONAL BOARD FOR RESPIRATORY CARE (NBRC)–TYPE QUESTIONS

1. The most reliable and rapid method for confirming ETT placement during a cardiac arrest involves the use of which of the following?
   A. Lateral chest radiography
   B. Bilateral chest auscultation
   C. An esophageal detection device
   D. A color-change capnometric device

2. The most appropriate device to facilitate the intubation of a patient with an unstable neck is which of the following?
   A. TT
   B. Carlens' tube
   C. Fiberoptic bronchoscope
   D. LMA

3. The device that allows visualization of the larynx without requiring alignment of the various axes of the airways is which of the following?
   A. Bullard laryngoscope
   B. Retrograde wire
   C. Laryngoscope
   D. LMA

4. A patient with a TT requires continuous mechanical ventilation and is frustrated with the fact that he is unable to speak. The RT should recommend the use of which of the following speaking devices?
   A. Fenestrated tracheostomy tube
   B. Olympic Medical
   C. Pitt speaking TT
   D. Passy-Muir valve

5. A patient sustained trauma to the right chest. The patient has developed right-sided pulmonary contusion and requires intubation. The most appropriate type of artificial airway to use is which of the following?
   A. LMA
   B. Combitube
   C. Double-lumen tube
   D. RAE tube

6. An intubated patient being manually ventilated continues to have a low partial pressure of arterial oxygen (Pao_2) despite the oxygen flow being 15 L/min. The RT should check which of the following for proper function?
   1. Pop-off valve
   2. Safety air inlet
   3. Safety oxygen outlet
   4. Reservoir bag connection
   A. 1, 2, and 4
   B. 2, 3, and 4
   C. 1, 2, and 3
   D. 1, 3, and 4

7. During mask ventilation the patient's chest is not rising. The most appropriate immediate action for the RT to take is which of the following?
   A. Reposition the mask.
   B. Open the pop-off valve.
   C. Change resuscitator bags.
   D. Increase the flow to the reservoir.

8. During oral endotracheal intubation, the most appropriate head and neck position for a patient is which of the following?
   A. In a flat position
   B. In the "sniffing" position
   C. In a chin-down position
   D. With a maximally flexed back

9. The airway examination component that suggests that a patient may have a difficult airway is which of the following?
   A. Flat palate
   B. Mallampati class III
   C. Interincisor distance of 4 cm
   D. Four-finger thyromental distance

10. A bystander has established unresponsiveness in a person who has collapsed suddenly. Which of the following is the most appropriate action at this time?
    A. Administer mouth-to-mouth resuscitation.
    B. Administer chest compressions at a rate of 100/min.
    C. Perform an abdominal thrust (Heimlich maneuver).
    D. Open the airway and wait for medical personnel to arrive.

Chapter **5** Airway Management Devices and Advanced Cardiac Life Support

6 Humidity and Aerosol Therapy

LEARNING OBJECTIVES

Upon completion of this chapter, you will be able to:

1. Differentiate humidity from aerosol.
2. Differentiate the roles of humidity and aerosol in respiratory care.
3. Describe the mechanisms of humidification.
4. Describe the natural physiologic humidification process throughout the respiratory tract.
5. Identify indications, contraindications, and hazards associated with humidity therapy.
6. Describe how various types of humidifiers work.
7. Compare and contrast low-flow and high-flow humidifiers.
8. Explain the importance of monitoring and maintaining humidity therapy.
9. Describe the physical characteristics of an aerosol.
10. Discuss factors that influence aerosol deposition.
11. Describe the therapeutic indications for aerosol therapy.
12. Identify special considerations for administering aerosol therapy.
13. Determine the optimal technique for administering aerosol: small-volume nebulizer, large-volume nebulizer, pressurized metered-dose inhaler, or dry powder inhaler.
14. Explain how pneumatic, ultrasonic, and vibrating mesh aerosol generators work.
15. Discuss criteria for device selection.
16. Describe how each type of device should be set up, used, and maintained.

"It's not the heat; it's the humidity."
Proverb

ACHIEVING THE OBJECTIVES

1. Differentiate humidity from aerosol. (IIIB8)

1A. What is humidity?

individual molecules
in a vapor gaseous
state

1B. What does a vapor consist of?

individual free molecules
of substance that exist below its
critical temp.

1C. What is an aerosol?

a suspension of solid or
liquid particles in a
gas. They occur in nature

1D. How does humidity differ from aerosol?

Humidity is composed of only
water whereas aerosol can be
water or another substance

1E. What is humidity used for in respiratory care?

used to maintain normal
physiologic conditions
for the airway

1F. Why is humidity therapy necessary when supplemental oxygen is administered?

Supplemental o₂ is cold & dry
& can cause drying of the airway &
reduce with moisture

1G. What is aerosol therapy used for in respiratory care?

They can be used bland or
medicated

Think About This:
What types of aerosols are you exposed to every day?

2. Differentiate the roles of humidity and aerosol in respiratory care. (IIIB8)

2A. What is the primary goal of humidity in respiratory care?

_____

2B. What is it that necessitates humidity when supplemental oxygen is being delivered?

_____

2C. List the roles that bland aerosol therapy has in respiratory care.

_____

2D. What is the goal of aerosol drug therapy?

_____

Think About This:
Why do you get thirsty in the desert?

3. Describe the mechanisms of humidification. (IIIB8)

3A. How is inhaled air humidified naturally?

_____

3B. What is another name for humidity?

_____

3C. When a gas is warmed, what happens to its capacity to hold water?

_____

3D. Name two ways in which humidity is described.

_____

Chapter **6 Humidity and Aerosol Therapy**

3E. Explain the two ways to describe humidity.

_____

_____

_____

_____

_____

3F. What would a hygrometer reading be if the relative humidity is 85% at 25° C? (*Hint: use Table 6-1 in the textbook.*)

_____

_____

_____

3G. What is the relative humidity when the hygrometer reading is 15.4 mg/L at 29° C?

_____

3H. What is the absolute humidity at body temperature when saturation is 100%?

_____

3I. List three types of active humidifiers.

_____

_____

_____

3J. Give an example of a passive humidifier.

_____

Think About This:

What is the perfect humidity level for your home?

4. Describe the natural physiologic humidification process throughout the respiratory tract. (IIIB8)

4A. During what part of the breath cycle do the upper airways add heat and humidity?

_____

_____

4B. During what part of the breath cycle is water reclaimed by the upper airways?

_____

_____

4C. What part of the nose increases the contact time between the inspired air and the nasal mucosa?

_____

_____

4D. Why does cold weather cause "runny" noses?

_____

_____

_____

_____

_____

4E. Why does a "stuffy" nose cause a dry mouth?

_____

_____

_____

Questions 4F through 4I refer to Figure 6-1.

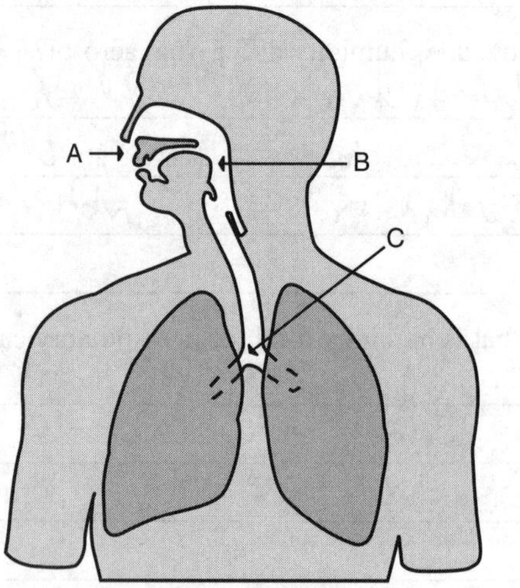

FIGURE 6-1

4F. Under ambient conditions, how much humidity is added to the inhaled air between point *A* and point *B*?

_____

_____

4G. Under ambient conditions, how much humidity is added to the inhaled air between point *B* and point *C*?

_____

_____

4H. At what point is the absolute humidity always 44 mg/L and the temperature 37° C?

_____

_____

_____

4I. At what point is the isothermic saturation boundary (ISB)?

_____

_____

Think About This:

Does the ISB change positions when a person is nose-breathing in the desert?

5. Identify indications, contraindications, and hazards associated with humidity therapy. (IIIB8)

5A. The presence of what seven clinical signs and symptoms, along with the administration of dry medical gas, are indications for humidity therapy?

Atelectasis, dry non productive cough, increased airway resistance, infection, increased WOB, pain, thick dehydrated secretions

5B. Why is heated humidity appropriate for patients who are hypothermic?

raises core temp back to normal

_____

_____

5C. Why is heated humidity helpful during cold-induced asthma attacks?

helps ↓ inflammation

_____

5D. Regardless of whether a patient with bypassed upper airways is breathing spontaneously or receiving mechanical ventilation, why should humidity therapy be administered?

When the upper airway is bypassed we do not have natural humidification system of humidity is not added the trachea can become damaged

_____

5E. Name the seven indications for the use of cool humidified gas (bland aerosol) as mentioned in the American Association for Respiratory Care (AARC) Clinical Practice Guideline (CPG) for Bland Aerosol Administration.

- upper airway edema
- laryngotracheobronchitis
- subglottic edema
- post extubation edema
- postoperative mgmt
- presence of a bypassed upper airway
- need for sputum specimens or mobilization of secretions

5F. List the 13 hazards and complications associated with the use of heated humidifiers. (See AARC CPG: Humidification During Mechanical Ventilation, http://www.aarc.org.)

- High flow rates during disconnect might aerosolize contaminated condensate.
- underhydration & mucus impaction.
- increased WOB
- elevated airway pressure caused by condensation
- patient-ventilator dyssynchrony & improper ventilation dyssynchrony
- hyperventilation & gas trapping
- hypothermia - burns
- electrical shock - airway burns. - increased WOB caused by mucus plugging
- unintended tracheal ____
- inadvertent tracheal lavage

5G. List the five contraindications for the use of heat and moisture exchangers (HMEs).

_____

_____

_____

_____

_____

_____

5H. What are the two contraindications for the use of bland aerosol administration? (See AARC CPG: Bland Aerosol Administration, http://www.aarc.org.)

_____

_____

Think About This:

What humidity level is optimum for individuals with chronic obstructive pulmonary disease (COPD)?

6. Describe how various types of humidifiers work. (IIA3)

Questions 6A and 6B refer to Figure 6-2.

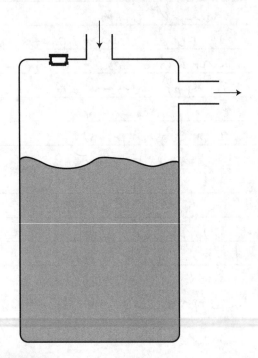

FIGURE 6-2
(Redrawn from Fink J, Cohen N: Humidity and aerosols. In Eubanks DH, Bone RC: *Principles and applications of cardiorespiratory care equipment*, St Louis, 1994, Mosby.)

6A. What type of humidifier is shown in Figure 6-2?

_____

6B. How does the humidifier shown in Figure 6-2 add humidity to the gas?

_____

_____

6C. What type of humidifier brings the gas under the surface of the water?

_____

_____

Questions 6D and 6E refer to Figure 6-3.

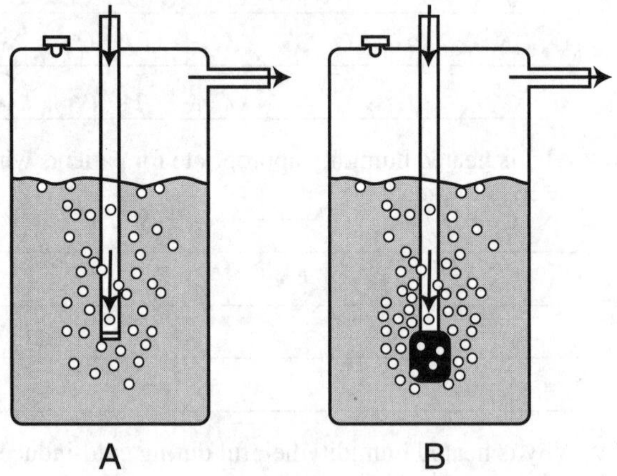

A   B

FIGURE 6-3

6D. What is the difference between the two humidifiers shown in Figure 6-3; which one is more efficient?

_____

_____

_____

6E. What would happen to one of the humidifiers shown in Figure 6-3 if the oxygen tubing connected to it becomes caught in the bed rails and is crimped off?

_____

_____

_____

_____

6F. What does adding heat do to a humidifier?

_____

_____

6G. Describe how a wick humidifier operates.

_____

_____

_____

_____

_____

_____

_____

6H. How does a membrane-type humidifier operate?

_____

_____

_____

_____

_____

6I. How does a large-volume jet nebulizer add humidity to a gas?

_____

_____

_____

_____

_____

6J. How does an ultrasonic nebulizer operate?

_____

_____

_____

_____

_____

_____

6K. How can particle size and aerosol density be altered on an ultrasonic nebulizer?

_____

_____

_____

_____

6L. Explain the operation of a generic HME.

_____

_____

_____

6M. Explain the operation of a condenser HME.

_____

_____

_____

_____

_____

_____

6N. How does a hygroscopic condenser HME operate?

_____

_____

_____

_____

_____

6O. Explain the operation of a hygroscopic HME filter.

_____

_____

_____

_____

_____

Think About This:
What are the different types of room humidifiers?

7. Compare and contrast low-flow and high-flow humidifiers. (IIA3)

7A. What is the maximum flow rate that should be used with a low-flow humidifier?

_____

_____

7B. Name a low-flow humidifier.

_____

_____

7C. What type of oxygen devices are used with low-flow humidifiers?

_____

_____

7D. Why shouldn't a low-flow humidifier be used with a patient who has a bypassed airway?

_____

_____

_____

_____

_____

_____

_____

7E. What are the two main structural differences between a low-flow humidifier and a high-flow humidifier?

_____

_____

_____

7F. What flow rates can a high-flow humidifier handle?

_____

_____

7G. Label the following humidifiers as either low-flow or high-flow humidifiers.

1. Bubble humidifier:

_____

_____

2. Heated passover humidifier:

_____

_____

3. HME:

_____

_____

4. Passover humidifier on a nasal cannula:

_____

_____

5. Diffuser bubble humidifier:

_____

_____

6. Large-volume nebulizer:

_____

_____

7. Ultrasonic nebulizer:

_____

_____

Think About This:
Are room humidifiers high-flow or low-flow humidifiers?

8. Explain the importance of monitoring and maintaining humidity therapy. (IIIB8)

8A. Why is inspecting the water level of a bubble humidifier important?

_____

_____

_____

_____

8B. Compare the humidity output of a bubble humidifier at 4 L/min versus one at 10 L/min.

_____

_____

_____

_____

8C. Why is inspecting the ventilator circuit for condensation important when a heated humidification system is being used?

_____

_____

_____

_____

_____

_____

_____

8D. List and explain four ways to reduce the collection of condensation in a ventilator circuit.

_____

_____

_____

_____

_____

_____

_____

8E. What device may be used to accurately and reliably ensure that patients are receiving gas at the expected temperature and humidity level?

_____

_____

8F. What factors should a respiratory therapist (RT) monitor when using an HME during mechanical ventilation of a patient?

_____

_____

_____

_____

_____

8G. According to the AARC, what factors should an RT monitor when a patient is receiving humidity therapy via a large-volume nebulizer?

_____

_____

_____

_____

_____

Think About This:

What causes ground fog?

9. Describe the physical characteristics of an aerosol. (IIIB8)

9A. Aerosols consisting of particles of a similar size are known as

_____

_____.

9B. Aerosols containing particles of many different sizes are known as

_____

_____.

9C. The average aerosol particle size expressed by the measure of central tendency for cascade impaction is known as _____;

for laser diffraction it is called

_____.

9D. As the geometric standard deviation becomes greater, what happens to the range of particle sizes?

_____

_____

_____

9E. What size particles usually remain in suspension and will be cleared with exhaled gas?

_____

_____

9F. What characteristic causes aerosol particles to increase in size as they age?

_____

_____

9G. What characteristic causes aerosol particles to decrease in size as they age?

_____

_____

Think About This:

How much aerosol are you exposed to during a normal day?

10. Discuss factors that influence aerosol deposition. (IIID5a)

10A. How does aerosol particle size influence its deposition?

function of particle size & velocity increases 7 larger size d velocities

10B. What is the primary mechanism for deposition of particles in the 1- to 5-micrometer range?

sedmentation

_____

_____

_____

_____

10C. What is the primary mechanism for the deposition of aerosol particles that are less than 3 micrometers in size?

diffusion

_____

10D. List five patient factors that influence the deposition of aerosols.

size & VT

shape

Age

particles

_____

_____

10E. What size particles have maximum deposition in the lungs?

.40

_____

Questions 10F and 10H refer to Figure 6-4.

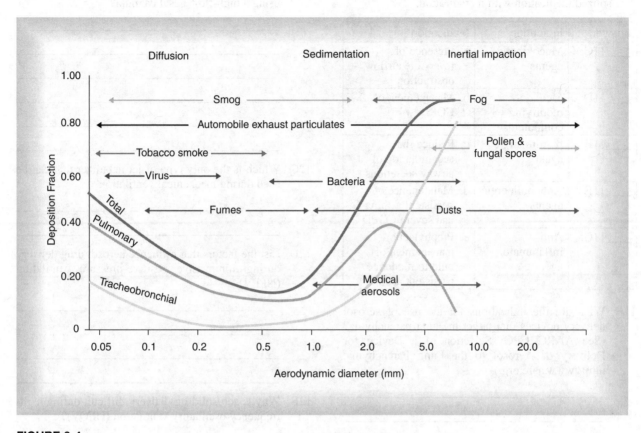

FIGURE 6-4
(From Kacmarek RL, Stoller JK, Heuer AJ: *Egan's fundamentals of respiratory care*, ed 10, St Louis, 2013, Mosby.)

10F. What five common aerosols are primarily deposited in the lungs by sedimentation?

_____

_____

_____

_____

_____

10G. Inertial impaction is the sole cause of deposition in the lungs for

_____

_____.

10H. Viruses are primarily deposited in the lungs by what mechanism?

_____

_____

Think About This:

What types of particles will high-efficiency particulate air (HEPA) filters remove from the air?

11. Describe the therapeutic indications for aerosol therapy. (IIID5a)

11A. State the goal of medical aerosol therapy.

_____

_____

_____

_____

11B. Why is administering medications by aerosol beneficial to patients with pulmonary disorders?

_____

_____

_____

_____

71

For questions 11C through 11G, match the aerosolized medication with its indication.

Answer	Indication	Medication
____11C.	Mucokinetic agents	a. Presence of reversible airflow obstruction
____11D.	Mediator-modifying compounds	b. Management of COPD
____11E.	β-Adrenergic agent	c. Reduce the accumulation of airway secretions
____11F.	Anticholinergic agents	d. Maintenance of persistent asthma and severe COPD
____11G.	Anti-inflammatory agent	e. Prophylactic management of mild to moderate persistent asthma

11H. What are the indications for the use of aerosol delivery devices that target the lung parenchyma? (See AARC CPG: Selection of a Device for Delivery of Aerosol to the Lung Parenchyma, http://www.aarc.org.)

_____

_____

11I. What are the seven indications for bland aerosol therapy? (See AARC CPG: Bland Aerosol Administration, http://www.aarc.org.)

_____

_____

_____

_____

_____

Think About This:

Observe someone you know using a pressurized meter-dosed inhaler (MDI). Does he or she use it properly?

12. Identify special considerations for administering aerosol therapy. (IIID5a, IIIE6, IIIE11)

12A. Why is the "blow-by" technique for delivering aerosol to infants and young children not a good delivery option?

_____

_____

12B. What is recommended to optimize aerosol delivery using a high-flow nasal cannula?

_____

_____

_____

_____

_____

_____

12C. Which is the only type of jet nebulizer that can be used during mechanical ventilation?

_____

_____

12D. List the factors that influence aerosol drug delivery during noninvasive positive-pressure ventilation (NPPV).

_____

_____

_____

_____

12E. Why is aerosol drug delivery difficult during high-frequency oscillatory ventilation (HFOV)?

_____

_____

12F. What type of aerosol delivery device produces the greatest amount of secondhand aerosol?

_____

_____

_____

12G. Why are special small-volume nebulizers (SVNs) (e.g., Respirgard II) used to deliver aerosolized pentamidine?

_____

_____

_____

_____

12H. What other aerosolized medication is associated with health risks to health care providers?

_____

_____

12I. List the health risks that are associated with administration of pentamidine and ribavirin.

_____

_____

_____

12J. What other environmental precautions should be taken when ribavirin or pentamidine is administered?

_____

_____

_____

_____

_____

_____

12K. A patient in the emergency department is suspected of having active tuberculosis and needs to have an aerosol treatment. How should this treatment be administered?

_____

_____

_____

_____

_____

12L. How should the filters and nebulizer used in treatments with pentamidine and ribavirin be disposed of?

_____

_____

_____

_____

Think About This:

What other types of medications can be aerosolized?

13. Determine the optimal technique for administering aerosol: small-volume nebulizer (SVN), large-volume nebulizer, pressurized metered-dose inhaler. (IIA4, IIID5a, IIID5b)

13A. What should the RT set the flow rate at for a pneumatic SVN?

_____

_____

13B. The SVNs that use electrical or battery power are

_____

_____.

13C. What is the most effective position for a patient taking a treatment with an SVN?

_____

_____

13D. Describe the appropriate breathing pattern that should be used during SVN treatment.

_____

_____

13E. Where should an SVN be placed when used during mechanical ventilation?

_____

_____

13F. What ventilator parameters need to be adjusted when an SVN is being used with mechanical ventilation?

_____

_____

_____

_____

13G. What type of SVN can aerosolize medication without increasing the patient's tidal volume?

_____

_____

13H. What patient interface should be used with continuous bronchodilator therapy through a large-volume nebulizer?

_____

_____

13I. When should a pressurized metered-dose inhaler (MDI) be primed?

_____

_____

13J. What technique may be used as an alternative to placing the mouthpiece of an MDI into the mouth?

_____

_____

_____

_____

13K. How long should the breath be held after an MDI actuation?

_____

_____

13L. How much time should elapse between actuations from an MDI?

_____

_____

13M. At what point during the breathing cycle should an MDI be actuated?

_____

_____

13N. Describe the appropriate breathing pattern for MDI use.

_____

_____

_____

13O. What technique should be used if a breath hold is not possible when a patient is using an MDI with a valved holding chamber?

_____

_____

_____

_____

_____

13P. What is the most critical factor in the use of a DPI?

_____

_____

13Q. What types of patients would not be able to use a DPI?

_____

_____

Think About This:

Which aerosol delivery device is ideal?

14. Explain how pneumatic, ultrasonic, and vibrating mesh aerosol generators work. (IIA4)

Questions 14A through 14F refer to Figure 6-5.

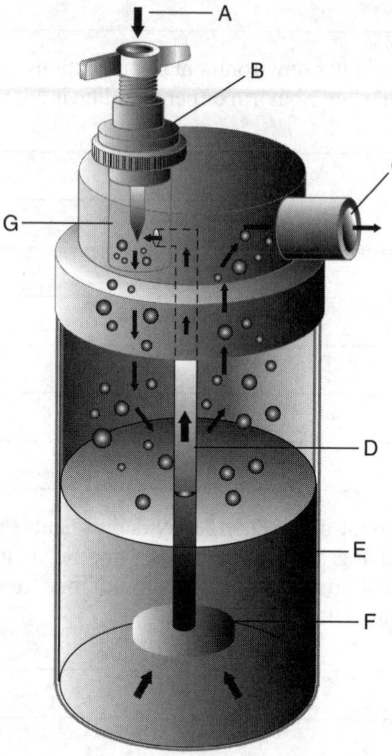

FIGURE 6-5
(From Kacmarek RL, Stoller JK, Heuer AJ: *Egan's fundamentals of respiratory care*, ed 10, St Louis, 2013, Mosby.)

14A. What type of device is shown in Figure 6-5?

_____

_____

14B. Label Figure 6-5.

A. _____

B. _____

C. _____

D. _____

E. _____

F. _____

G. _____

14C. How does the device in Figure 6-5 create aerosol particles?

_____

_____

_____

_____

_____

_____

_____

_____

14D. What flow rate should be used to operate the device in Figure 6-5?

_____

_____

14E. What is the total water output of the device in Figure 6-5 when unheated?

_____

_____

14F. What is the total water output of the device in Figure 6-5 when heated?

_____

_____

Questions 14G through 14M refer to Figure 6-6.

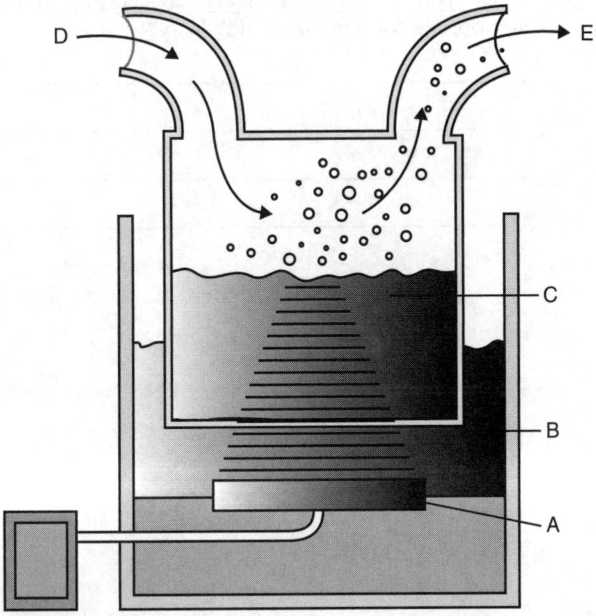

FIGURE 6-6
(From Kacmarek RL, Stoller JK, Heuer AJ: *Egan's fundamentals of respiratory care*, ed 10, St Louis, 2013, Mosby.)

14G. What type of device is shown in Figure 6-6?

_____

_____

14H. Label Figure 6-6.

A. _____

B. _____

C. _____

D. _____

E. _____

14I. How does the device in Figure 6-6 create aerosol particles?

_____

_____

_____

_____

_____

_____

_____

_____

14J. On the device in Figure 6-6, particle size is dictated by

_____

_____.

14K. The rate of aerosol production by the device in Figure 6-6 is directly related to

_____

_____.

14L. What do the flow and amplitude settings for the equipment shown in Figure 6-6 determine?

_____

_____

14M. What is the maximum total water output for the device in Figure 6-6?

_____

_____

75

14N. How does a vibrating mesh nebulizer create an aerosol?

_____

_____

_____

_____

14O. What is the difference between a passive vibrating mesh nebulizer and an active vibrating mesh nebulizer?

_____

_____

_____

_____

_____

_____

_____

Think About This:

Do pets have a need for nebulizers?

15. Discuss criteria for device selection. (IIA4, IIA23, IIIC3, IIID5a)

15A. What are the five factors that should be considered when selecting the appropriate aerosol delivery device for a given patient?

_____

_____

_____

_____

15B. An alert and oriented elderly patient with arthritis requires the use of an aerosol delivery device at home for a bronchodilator; what are the pros and cons of each delivery device?

_____

_____

_____

_____

_____

_____

_____

_____

_____

_____

15C. A patient with asthma arrives at the emergency department in respiratory distress. Which type of delivery system is most appropriate to treat this patient with an aerosolized bronchodilator? Why?

_____

_____

_____

_____

_____

_____

_____

15D. What types of aerosol delivery device(s) are most appropriate for a young child? Why?

_____

_____

_____

15E. An RT has decided that a 6-year-old, actively cooperative child is able to use an MDI with a valved holding chamber (VHC) to take her aerosolized medication. The child's parents, however, insist on an SVN with a compressor. What is the most appropriate action for the RT to take? Why?

_____

_____

_____

_____

_____

15F. A patient receiving mechanical ventilation requires an aerosolized medication. What are the most appropriate aerosol delivery devices for this situation? Why?

_____

_____

_____

_____

_____

_____

15G. What device should be used to deliver ribavirin to a child with respiratory syncytial virus?

_____

_____

15H. Name three brands of SVNs that are made to deliver aerosolized pentamidine.

_____

_____

_____

Think About This:

How do aerosol deposition and dispersion change in an environment with altered gravity?

16. Describe how each type of device should be set up, used, and maintained. (IIA4, IIA23, IIA24)

16A. When should an MDI be primed?

_____

_____

_____

_____

16B. What is the proper technique for priming an MDI?

_____

_____

16C. When should the MDI open-mouth technique not be used?

_____

_____

16D. Describe how an MDI should be cleaned.

_____

_____

_____

_____

16E. When should an MDI be discarded?

_____

_____

_____

16F. How should a VHC be maintained?

_____

_____

16G. What is the procedure for priming a new dry powder inhaler (DPI)?

_____

_____

_____

_____

16H. What are the steps for the use of a DPI?

_____

_____

_____

_____

_____

_____

_____

_____

_____

_____

16I. How should a DPI be stored?

_____

_____

_____

16J. What is the technique for the use of a vibrating mesh or ultrasonic nebulizer?

_____

_____

_____

_____

16K. How should a nebulizer be maintained at home after each use?

_____

_____

_____

16L. How often should a home nebulizer be disinfected?

_____

_____

16M. What is the procedure for disinfecting a home nebulizer?

_____

_____

_____

_____

16N. Give three examples of disinfectant options for the home nebulizer.

_____

_____

_____

_____

_____

16O. How should a ventilator be set up for the administration of pressurized MDI (pMDI) in the ventilator circuit?

_____

_____

_____

_____

_____

_____

16P. How long should the RT wait between actuations when delivering medication via a pressurized MDI in a ventilator circuit?

_____

_____

Think About This:
Does asthma occur in pets and other animals?

NATIONAL BOARD FOR RESPIRATORY CARE (NBRC)–TYPE QUESTIONS

1. What happens at the ISB?
   A. No more cilia exist.
   B. Turbulent convection occurs.
   C. Inspired gas reaches body humidity.
   D. The largest humidity deficit exists.

2. Water moves up the "wick" of a wick humidifier because of which of the following?
   A. Venturi principle
   B. Bernoulli principle
   C. Capillary action
   D. Boyle's law

3. The type of humidifier that uses a low thermal conductivity condensing element is which of the following?
   A. Wick humidifier
   B. Bubble humidifier
   C. Ultrasonic nebulizer
   D. Hygroscopic HME

4. What is the relative humidity when the absolute humidity is 10 mg H_2O/L and the capacity is 18 mg H_2O/L?
   A. 23%
   B. 38%
   C. 41%
   D. 55%

5. A patient is receiving oxygen therapy via a simple mask at a flow of 15 L/min with a bubble humidifier. A clinical assessment reveals a nonproductive cough. The patient is reporting a dry mouth, nose, and throat. The most appropriate action(s) to take include which of the following?
   1. Decrease the oxygen flow rate to the simple mask to 10 L/min.
   2. Replace the apparatus with an SVN.
   3. Suggest an aerosol treatment with a mucolytic agent.
   4. Check the humidifier water level.
   A. 4 only
   B. 2 only
   C. 1 and 4 only
   D. 2 and 3 only

6. While checking a patient who is receiving oxygen, an RT hears a high-pitched whistle coming from the bubble humidifier. The most probable cause of the problem is which of the following?
   A. The oxygen tubing is kinked.
   B. The humidifier is overheated.
   C. Nasal prongs are not in place.
   D. Water level in the humidifier is low.

7. A heated humidifier unit has a water temperature of 40° C. The humidified gas is traveling through large-bore tubing to the patient. Which of the following statements are true?
   1. Condensation will occur.
   2. The gas will remain saturated.
   3. The relative humidity will increase.
   4. The gas will warm and expand as it travels to the patient.
   A. 1 and 2 only
   B. 2 and 3 only
   C. 3 and 4 only
   D. 1 and 4 only

8. Clinical signs and symptoms of inadequate airway humidification include all of the following **EXCEPT**
   A. Atelectasis
   B. Substernal pain
   C. Productive cough
   D. Increased work of breathing

9. Which of the following statements are true concerning bubble humidifiers?
   1. At 4 L/min the absolute humidity is approximately 30 mg/L.
   2. They are more efficient at flows greater than 5 L/min.
   3. At best, a bubble humidifier can deliver 20% relative humidity at body temperature and pressure saturated.
   4. The pressure-relief alarm sounds when pressure in the unit exceeds 2 psi.
   A. 1 and 2 only
   B. 2 and 3 only
   C. 3 and 4 only
   D. 1 and 4 only

10. The primary mechanism for deposition of small particles of less than 3 micrometers is which of the following?
    A. Sedimentation
    B. Inertial impaction
    C. Brownian motion
    D. Monodispersion

79

11. A hypothermic patient with a bypassed airway requires humidification. Which of the following humidifiers would be most appropriate for this situation?
    1. Wick humidifier
    2. Bubble humidifier
    3. Large-volume nebulizer
    4. Hygroscopic HME
       A. 1 and 3 only
       B. 2 and 3 only
       C. 1, 3, and 4 only
       D. 2, 3, and 4 only

12. The RT should coach a patient to breathe in which of the following patterns for particle deposition in the lower airways?
    1. Inhale slowly.
    2. Inhale rapidly.
    3. Inhale deeply through the nose.
    4. Use a mouthpiece instead of a mask.
    5. Take occasional deep breaths.
       A. 2 and 3 only
       B. 2 and 5 only
       C. 1, 3, and 5 only
       D. 1, 4, and 5 only

13. Bland aerosol therapy is delivered most appropriately to a patient with a tracheostomy tube through which of the following methods?
    A. Humidifier, oxygen tubing, and a nasal cannula
    B. Large-volume nebulizer, large-bore tubing, and a Briggs adapter
    C. Large-volume nebulizer, large-bore tubing, and a tracheostomy collar
    D. SVN, oxygen tubing, and a large-volume nebulizer

14. Which of the following devices is used most commonly to deliver continuous aerosol with oxygen to a patient with a tracheostomy?
    A. Vibrating mesh nebulizer
    B. Pneumatic jet nebulizer
    C. HME
    D. Small-particle aerosol generator

15. The RT administers a bronchodilator with a pMDI to a patient receiving mechanical ventilation. Which of the following are correct regarding this procedure?
    1. The HME should be removed.
    2. The adapter should be placed in the inspiratory limb.
    3. The peak inspiratory flow should be increased as tolerated.
    4. At least 15 seconds should be allowed between actuations.
       A. 1 and 2 only
       B. 2 and 3 only
       C. 1, 2, and 3 only
       D. 1, 2, and 4 only

16. The device selected for the administration of pharmacologically active aerosol to the lower airway should produce particles with a mass median aerodynamic diameter range of
    A. 0.5 to 1 micrometers.
    B. 1 to 5 micrometers.
    C. 6 to 10 micrometers.
    D. 10 to 20 micrometers.

17. A patient with asthma and severe bronchospasm is not responding to intermittent SVN treatments with a β-adrenergic bronchodilator. The appropriate recommendation for this patient is to switch to which of the following?
    A. Dry powder inhaler (DPI) bronchodilator
    B. Continuous bronchodilator therapy
    C. Continuous nebulized bland aerosol
    D. MDI bronchodilator with a VHC

18. To prevent the hazards of contact with ribavirin, caregivers must wear which of the following?
    1. Gown
    2. Gloves
    3. Goggles
    4. HEPA mask
       A. 3 and 4 only
       B. 1 and 2 only
       C. 2, 3, and 4 only
       D. 1, 2, 3, and 4

19. Aerosol deposition in the lungs will be increased according to all of the following **EXCEPT**
    A. Breath-holding.
    B. Decreased tidal volume.
    C. Decreased respiratory rate.
    D. Increased inspiratory to expiratory time.

20. A patient is set up on a 35% aerosol mask. Several hours later, an oxygen analyzer is placed in the circuit and its reading is 60%, but the large-volume nebulizer setting remains at 35%. The most appropriate action is which of the following?
    A. Shorten the aerosol tubing.
    B. Increase the nebulizer flow.
    C. Decrease the nebulizer flow.
    D. Drain the water from the aerosol tubing.

Lung Expansion Therapy Devices

Upon completion of this chapter, you will be able to:
1. Compare volume-displacement and flow-dependent incentive spirometers.
2. Describe two types of machines used to administer intermittent positive pressure breathing therapy.
3. Discuss how expiratory positive airway pressure, continuous positive airway pressure, and positive expiratory pressure therapies are used to mobilize secretions and treat atelectasis.
4. Identify the major components of pneumatically and electrically powered percussors.
5. Describe the theory of operation of four devices that enhance clearance of airway secretions by producing high-frequency oscillations to the lungs and chest wall.
6. Discuss how mechanical insufflation-exsufflation devices can enhance airway secretions in patients with respiratory muscle weakness or paralysis.

"Nothing in life is to be feared. It is only to be understood."
Marie Curie

ACHIEVING THE OBJECTIVES

1. Compare volume-displacement and flow-dependent incentive spirometers. (IIAI3, IIID1a)

1A. What is incentive spirometry?

_____

_____

1B. List three indications for incentive spirometry.

_____

_____

_____

_____

1C. Define sustained maximum inspiration (SMI).

_____

_____

_____

1D. How does a volume-displacement incentive spirometer operate?

_____

_____

_____

_____

1E. How does a flow-dependent incentive spirometer operate?

_____

_____

_____

1F. How is volume displacement achieved with a flow-dependent incentive spirometer?

_____

_____

1G. An SMI should be how long?

_____

1H. A patient using a flow-dependent incentive spirometer holds an inspiratory flow of 900 mL/s for 1.5 seconds. The amount of volume inhaled by the patient during this maneuver is

_____

_____.

Think About This:
What types of breathing patterns can occur when a person is under stress?

2. Describe two types of machines used to administer intermittent positive pressure breathing (IPPB) therapy. (IIA11b, IIID2a)

2A. Define _intermittent positive pressure breathing (IPPB)_.

_____

_____

2B. List the indications for IPPB therapy.

_____

_____

_____

_____

_____

_____

_____

2C. What should be monitored during IPPB therapy?

_____

_____

_____

_____

_____

_____

2D. Which types of devices are used to deliver IPPB therapy?

_____

_____

82

Chapter **7** **Lung Expansion Therapy Devices**

2E. What types of IPPB devices does Puritan Bennett manufacture?

_____

_____

2F. Which Puritan Bennett IPPB devices could also be used to provide short-term ventilation for patients with apnea?

_____

_____

2G. Describe the IPPB devices mentioned in question 2F in terms of their phase variables.

_____

_____

2H. What types of IPPB devices does Bird manufacture?

_____

2I. What is the basic operational principle of the Bird IPPB devices?

_____

_____

2J. Describe the Bird IPPB devices in terms of their phase variables.

_____

_____

2K. Describe the Vortran-IPPB device in terms of its phase variables.

_____

_____

_____

2L. What is the primary advantage of the Vortran-IPPB device?

_____

_____

Think About This:
Why is IPPB therapy so controversial?

3. Discuss how expiratory positive airway pressure (EPAP), continuous positive airway pressure (CPAP), and positive expiratory pressure (PEP) therapies are used to mobilize secretions and treat atelectasis. (IIA14c)

3A. What are four indications for the use of positive airway pressure devices?

_____

_____

_____

_____

_____.

3B. How does CPAP operate?

_____

_____

3C. Describe how EPAP works.

_____

_____

_____

_____

3D. Describe how PEP operates.

_____

_____

_____

3E. How does PEP therapy prevent atelectasis?

_____

_____

_____

3F. What other therapy may be administered simultaneously using a PEP device?

_____

Think About This:
What do the pressure-time waveforms look like for EPAP and PEP?

4. Identify the major components of pneumatically and electrically powered percussors. (IIA14a)

4A. How do both electrically and pneumatically powered percussors clear airway secretions?

_____

_____

_____

_____

4B. How much gas pressure is necessary to power pneumatic percussors?

_____

_____

4C. What are the major components of a pneumatically powered percussor?

_____

_____

_____

_____

4D. What type of electrical current is necessary to power an electric percussor?

_____

_____

_____

4E. What major components are common to electrically powered percussors?

_____

_____

_____

4F. Which type or types of percussors can be used in home care?

_____

_____

Think About This:

Can you think of a household item that can be used to improvise a manual percussor?

5. Describe the theory of operation of four devices that enhance clearance of airway secretions by delivering high-frequency oscillations to the lungs and chest wall. (IIA14b)

5A. What factors are thought to enhance clearance of airway secretions by high-frequency oscillation devices?

_____

_____

_____

_____

_____

5B. Name the two devices that transmit high-frequency oscillation through the airway opening.

_____

_____

5C. Name the two devices that deliver high-frequency oscillation to the chest wall.

_____

_____

5D. Describe how the Percussionaire Intrapulmonary Percussive Ventilator (IPV-1) unit operates.

_____

_____

_____

_____

_____

_____

_____

_____

5E. What is the main advantage of the Acapella valve over the Flutter valve?

_____

_____

_____

5F. How many breaths should be exhaled through the Flutter valve or the Acapella valve?

_____

5G. Explain how the Vest airway clearance system operates.

_____

_____

_____

_____

_____

_____

5H. Explain the operation of the Hayek Oscillator.

_____

_____

_____

_____

_____

_____

_____

_____

Think About This:

How have chest physiotherapy devices improved the lives of individuals with cystic fibrosis?

6. Discuss how mechanical insufflation-exsufflation (MI-E) devices can enhance airway secretions in patients with respiratory muscle weakness or paralysis. (IIA14d)

6A. What is the purpose of the MI-E device?

_____

_____

_____

6B. How does the MI-E device (e.g., Respironics CoughAssist) operate?

_____

_____

_____

_____

_____

_____

_____

6C. For what disease process has the Respironics CoughAssist been shown to be most effective?

_____

_____

Think About This:

What could happen if a patient with emphysema used an MI-E device?

NATIONAL BOARD FOR RESPIRATORY CARE (NBRC)–TYPE QUESTIONS

1. Contraindications for incentive spirometry include which of the following?
   A. Post-thoracic surgery
   B. Vital capacity < 10 mL/kg
   C. Restrictive pulmonary disease
   D. Inspiratory capacity > predicted value

2. A patient reports that during incentive spirometry she becomes light-headed and dizzy and must stop the maneuver when this happens. The most probable cause is that the patient is
   A. Hypoventilating.
   B. Hyperventilating.
   C. Becoming fatigued.
   D. Having a bronchospasm.

3. Myasthenia gravis is causing a patient to have respiratory muscle weakness. This patient has a vital capacity of 5 mL/kg and is unable to cough effectively. What therapy would you recommend to help prevent pulmonary complications?
   A. Incentive spirometry
   B. Positive expiratory pressure
   C. Mechanical insufflation-exsufflation
   D. Intermittent positive pressure breathing (IPPB)

4. Which of the following IPPB machines is unable to provide short-term ventilatory support?
   A. Bird Mark 7
   B. Bird Mark 14
   C. Puritan Bennett AP-4
   D. Puritan Bennett PR-2

5. The therapy that mobilizes retained secretions, through the use of devices similar to continuous positive airway pressure (CPAP) resistors but that are less cumbersome, is
   A. Expiratory positive airway pressure (EPAP).
   B. IPPB.
   C. Intrapulmonary percussive ventilation (IPV).
   D. Positive expiratory pressure (PEP).

6. During a PEP therapy session, what directions should be given to the patient?
   A. "Stop after 20 to 30 breaths."
   B. "Place your lips into the mouthpiece."
   C. "Take a deep breath, then actively exhale."
   D. "Breathe normally through the mouthpiece."

7. What type of therapy is recommended to reduce air-trapping?
   A. IPV and chest physiotherapy
   B. IPPB and chest physiotherapy
   C. Positive airway pressure with PEP
   D. Positive airway pressure with CPAP of 15 cm H_2O

8. The type of adjunctive therapy that aids in the mobilization of airway secretions through high-frequency percussive breaths applied inside the patient's airways is known as what?
   A. IPV
   B. CPAP
   C. EPAP
   D. PEP

9. IPV mobilizes airway secretions by
   A. Generating subatmospheric pressure on inspiration, then expiratory resistance.
   B. Applying a positive pressure to a patient's airways throughout the respiratory cycle.
   C. Delivering high-frequency percussive breaths into the patient's airways.
   D. Applying expiratory resistance to exhaled flow from the patient.

10. To apply positive airway pressure to a manual resuscitator bag during patient transport, which of the following are most appropriate?
    1. Spring-loaded valve
    2. Underwater seal
    3. Magnetic valve
    4. Weighted ball
    A. 1 and 2 only
    B. 1 and 3 only
    C. 2 and 4 only
    D. 3 and 4 only

8 Assessment of Pulmonary Function

LEARNING OBJECTIVES

Upon completion of this chapter, you will be able to:

1. Identify three types of volume-collecting spirometers.
2. Explain the operational theory of thermal flowmeters.
3. Name three types of pneumotachometers.
4. Describe three types of body plethysmographs.
5. Discuss the American Thoracic Society/European Respiratory Society standards for lung function testing.
6. Compare the nitrogen washout and the helium dilution techniques for measuring functional residual capacity and residual volume.
7. Explain the operational theories of strain gauge, variable-inductance, and variable-capacitance pressure transducers.
8. Describe various conditions that interfere with the operation of impedance pneumographs.
9. List and describe measured and derived variables that are commonly used to assess respiratory mechanics.
10. Compare the operational principles of the two types of oxygen analyzers used in the clinical setting.
11. Describe two techniques for monitoring nitrogen oxides in the clinical setting.
12. Identify the components of a normal capnogram.
13. Assess an abnormal capnogram and suggest possible pathophysiologic processes that could contribute to the contour of the carbon dioxide waveform.
14. Compare closed-circuit and open-circuit indirect calorimeters.
15. Calculate energy expenditure by using measurements obtained during indirect calorimetry.
16. Explain how indirect calorimetry can be used to determine substrate utilization patterns in healthy individuals and in those with cardiopulmonary dysfunctions.

"The answer, my friend, is blowin' in the wind. The answer is blowin' in the wind."
Bob Dylan

ACHIEVING THE OBJECTIVES

1. Identify three types of volume-collecting spirometers. (IIA17)

1A. How do volume-collecting spirometers operate?

_____

_____

_____

1B. Identify the spirometer in Figure 8-1.

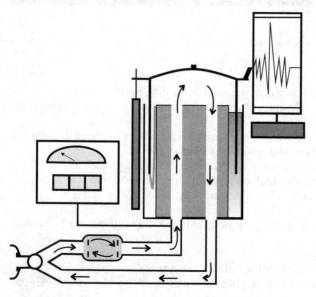

FIGURE 8-1
(From Mottram C: Ruppel's _Manual of pulmonary function testing_, ed 9, St Louis, 2013, Mosby.)

1C. Describe how the spirometer in Figure 8-1 operates.

_____

_____

_____

_____

_____

_____

_____

1D. Identify the spirometer in Figure 8-2.

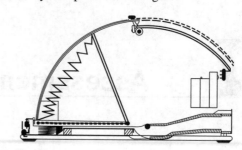

FIGURE 8-2
(Modified from Vitalograph, Shawnee Mission, Kansas.)

1E. Describe how the spirometer in Figure 8-2 operates.

_____

_____

_____

_____

_____

_____

_____

1F. What are the similarities and differences between the spirometers in Figure 8-1 and Figure 8-3?

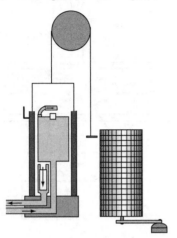

FIGURE 8-3
(Modified from Collins Medical, Braintree, Massachusetts.)

_____
_____
_____
_____
_____
_____
_____
_____
_____
_____
_____
_____
_____
_____
_____
_____

1G. Identify the spirometer in Figure 8-4.

_____

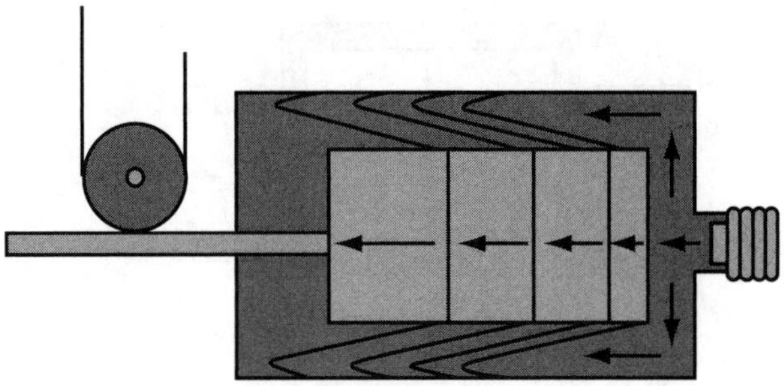

FIGURE 8-4
(From Datex-Ohmeda, Madison, Wisconsin.)

1H. Describe how the spirometer in Figure 8-4 operates.

_____
_____
_____
_____
_____
_____
_____
_____
_____

1I. What are the three types of volume-collecting spirometers?

_____
_____
_____

Think About This:
Are volume-collecting spirometers appropriate for use with young children and infants?

Chapter **8** **Assessment of Pulmonary Function**

2. Explain the operational theory of thermal flowmeters. (IIA17)

Questions 2A and 2B refer to Figure 8-5.

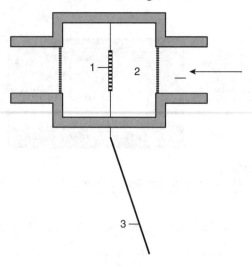

FIGURE 8-5

2A. Label Figure 8-5. (1) _____,

(2) _____, and

(3) _____.

2B. How does this type of flowmeter operate?

_____

_____

_____

_____

_____

2C. List four sources of errors that could interfere with the operation of a thermal flowmeter.

_____

_____

_____

_____

2D. What factors can affect the accuracy and precision of the flow measurement?

_____

_____

Think About This:

What other uses do hot-wire anemometers have?

3. Name three types of pneumotachometers. (IIA17)

Questions 3A through 3D refer to Figure 8-6.

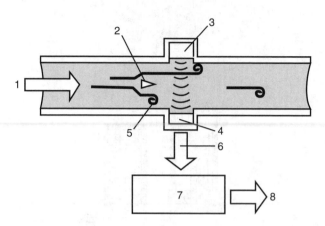

FIGURE 8-6
(Redrawn from Sullivan WJ, Peters GM, Enright PL: Pneumotachography: theory and clinical application, *Respir Care* 29:736, 1984.)

3A. What type of pneumotachometer is shown in Figure 8-6?

_____

_____

3B. Identify the parts labeled in Figure 8-6.

1.	
2.	
3.	
4.	
5.	
6.	
7.	
8.	

3C. How does the pneumotachograph shown in Figure 8-6 operate?

_____

_____

_____

_____

3D. Can the pneumotachograph shown in Figure 8-6 measure inspiratory and expiratory flow simultaneously?

_____

3E. What type of pneumotachograph measures flow by using a variable area and flexible obstruction for measuring flow as a function of the pressure differential generated by the obstruction?

_____

Questions 3F through 3H refer to Figure 8-7.

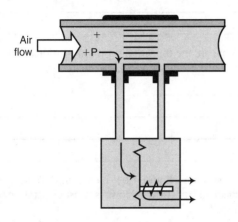

FIGURE 8-7
(Redrawn from Sullivan WJ, Peters GM, Enright PL: Pneumotachography: theory and clinical application, *Respir Care* 29:736, 1984.)

3F. What type of pneumotachograph is shown in Figure 8-7?

_____

_____

3G. How does the pneumotachograph in Figure 8-7 operate?

_____

_____

_____

_____

_____

3H. What is the purpose of having a heater in the pneumotachograph in Figure 8-7?

_____

_____

_____

3I. What type of pneumotachograph uses ceramic parallel channels instead of brass capillary tubes?

_____

_____

3J. What type of pneumotachograph uses a Monel screen as the main resistive component with a heating element?

_____

_____

3K. What type of pneumotachograph uses sound waves that are projected parallel to the flow of gas and also can be used to measure bidirectional flows?

_____

_____.

Think About This:
What use would a pneumotachograph have during speech therapy?

4. Describe three types of body plethysmographs. (IIIE7c)

4A. What measurements can be obtained with a body plethysmograph?

_____

_____

_____

_____

4B. What is the most common type of body plethysmograph?

_____

_____.

4C. How does the body plethysmograph in Question 4B operate?

_____

_____

_____

_____

_____

_____

_____

4D. How does a volume-displacement plethysmograph operate?

_____

_____

4E. To measure airflow changes during constant-pressure (volume-displacement) plethysmography, what equipment is incorporated into the body box?

_____

_____

Chapter **8** **Assessment of Pulmonary Function**

4F. What gas law is being applied during the use of body plethysmography?

_____

_____

Think About This:

How has body plethysmography been changed over the years to reduce claustrophobia?

5. Discuss the American Thoracic Society/ European Respiratory Society (ATS/ERS) standards for lung function testing. (IIC4, IIIE7a)

5A. The ATS/ERS documents provide guidance for which pulmonary function tests?

_____

_____

5B. Define the term *repeatability* as it relates to lung function testing.

_____

_____

_____

5C. What is the repeatability standard for forced expiratory volume in 1 second (FEV_1)?

_____

5D. What is the repeatability standard for peak expiratory flow (PEF)?

_____

_____

5E. How often should spirometry equipment be checked for volume and leaks?

_____

_____

5F. What methods are used to perform the volume and leak tests on spirometry equipment?

_____

_____

_____

5G. How frequently should the volume linearity of a spirometer be checked? How should this be accomplished?

_____

_____

_____

5H. What are the six diagnostic indications for spirometry according to ATS/ERS standards?

_____

_____

_____

_____

_____

5I. What are the four monitoring indications for spirometry according to ATS/ERS standards?

_____

_____

_____

_____

5J. How often should flow-measuring spirometers be checked for flow? How is this calibration check done?

_____

_____

_____

Think About This:

How does testing technique affect the ability to detect change in lung function?

6. Compare the nitrogen washout and the helium dilution techniques for measuring functional residual capacity (FRC) and residual volume. (IIIE7c)

6A. What gas is inhaled by the patient during a nitrogen washout test? _____

6B. What gas is inhaled by the patient during a helium dilution test? _____

6C. Describe how the nitrogen washout test enables you to measure FRC.

_____

_____

_____

_____

_____

_____

_____

_____

_____

_____

6D. Describe how the helium dilution test enables you to measure FRC.

_____

_____

_____

_____

_____

_____

_____

_____

_____

6E. What is an important consideration when measuring FRC with plethysmography as compared to inert gas techniques?

_____

_____

_____

_____

_____

Think About This:

What does the difference between a total lung capacity (TLC) measurement obtained by means of body plethysmography and a TLC measurement obtained by means of helium dilution represent?

7. Explain the operational theories of strain gauge, variable-inductance, and variable-capacitance pressure transducers. (IIA16)

7A. How does a strain gauge operate?

_____

_____

_____

_____

_____

_____

Questions 7B through 7D refer to Figure 8-8.

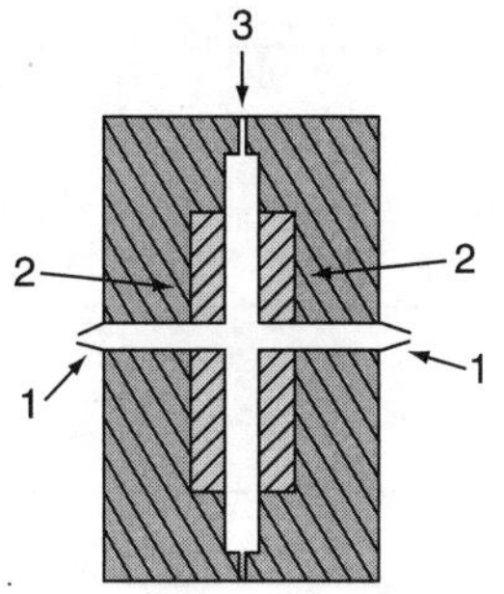

FIGURE 8-8
(Courtesy of Snow M: Instrumentation. In Clausen JL, ed: *Pulmonary function testing: guidelines and controversies*, New York, 1982, Academic Press.)

7B. What type of pressure transducer is shown in Figure 8-8?

_____

7C. Label Figure 8-8.

(1) _____

(2) _____

(3) _____

7D. Explain how the pressure transducer in Figure 8-8 operates.

_____

_____

_____

_____

_____

_____

Questions 7E through 7G refer to Figure 8-9.

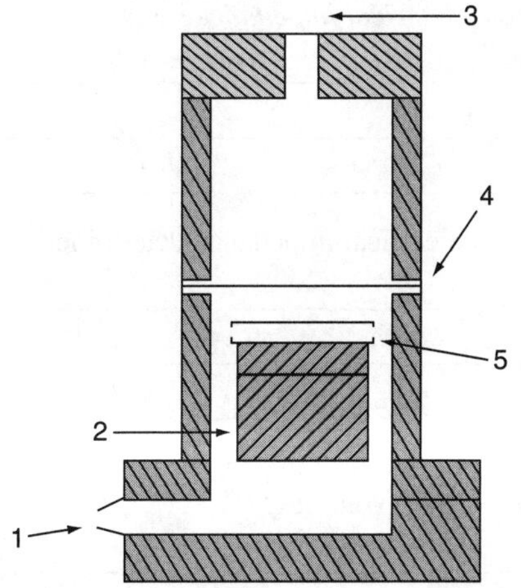

FIGURE 8-9
(Courtesy of Snow M: Instrumentation. In Clausen JL, ed: *Pulmonary function testing: guidelines and controversies*, New York, 1982, Academic Press.)

7E. What type of pressure transducer is shown in Figure 8-9?

_____

_____

7F. Label Figure 8-9.

(1) _____

(2) _____

(3) _____

(4) _____

(5) _____

7G. Explain the operation of the pressure transducer in Figure 8-9.

_____

_____

_____

_____

_____

_____

7H. Which two types of pressure transducers are most commonly used for measuring respiratory and cardiovascular pressures?

_____

_____

_____

Think About This:

In what other industries are pressure transducers used?

8. Describe various conditions that interfere with the operation of impedance pneumographs. (IIA17)

8A. Define *electrical impedance*.

_____

_____

_____

8B. How is electrical impedance determined?

_____

_____

_____

8C. How does electrical impedance facilitate the measurement of lung volumes?

_____

_____

_____

_____

_____

_____

_____

8D. What is the most common use for impedance pneumography?

_____

_____

8E. What alarms are incorporated into impedance pneumographs?

_____

_____

8F. Why is sensitivity of the impedance pneumographs an important setting?

_____

_____

_____

8G. What conditions can interfere with the proper operation of impedance pneumographs?

_____

_____

8H. How do these conditions interfere with impedance pneumographs?

_____

_____

_____

_____

_____

_____

_____

_____

8I. What other noninvasive method is used to measure respiratory function?

_____

_____

8J. How is respiratory impedance pneumography used clinically?

Think About This:

What other uses does impedance plethysmography have?

9. List and describe measured and derived variables that are commonly used to assess respiratory mechanics. (IA4, IA7b, IA7d, IB10n, IIIE7a, IIIE7b, IIIE7c)

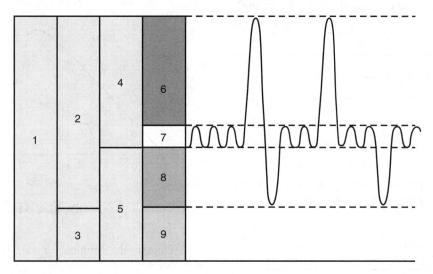

FIGURE 8-10
(From Comroe J: *The lung*, ed 3, Chicago, 1986, Mosby.)

9A. Label the volumes and capacities represented in Figure 8-10.

(1) _____   (6) _____

(2) _____   (7) _____

(3) _____   (8) _____

(4) _____   (9) _____

(5) _____

9B. What volume measurements are included in simple spirometry?

_____

_____

9C. What are the formulas for the ventilatory capacities calculated from simple spirometry?

_____

_____

_____

9D. What dynamic lung volumes can be measured with simple spirometry?

_____

_____

_____

9E. Compare simple spirometry with full lung-volume tests.

_____

_____

_____

_____

_____

_____

_____

9F. How are mechanically ventilated patients tested to assess their pulmonary progress and their ability to breathe spontaneously? What is the significance of the finding?

_____

_____

_____

_____

_____

_____

9G. What airway pressure measurements are usually performed on spontaneously breathing patients?

_____

_____

_____

_____

9H. How are these typical airway pressure measurements obtained?

_____

_____

_____

_____

_____

_____

9I. Define the two airway pressures that are most commonly measured while a patient is receiving mechanical ventilation.

_____

_____

_____

_____

_____

9J. What are the peak inspiratory pressure and the plateau pressure values in Figure 8-11?

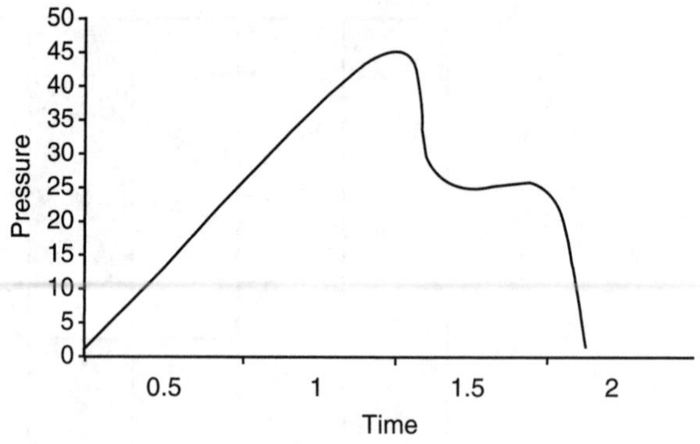

FIGURE 8-11

9K. What is the formula for calculating airway resistance?

_____

_____

9L. What information does airway resistance give about the status of the airways? What is the normal range of values for airway resistance?

_____

_____

_____

_____

9M. What is respiratory system compliance? What is the normal range of values for respiratory system compliance?

_____

_____

_____

_____

9N. What pulmonary conditions cause changes both in airway resistance and in respiratory system compliance?

_____

_____

_____

_____

_____

_____

Think About This:

How are respiratory mechanics assessed in newborns?

10. Compare the operational principles of the two types of oxygen analyzers used in the clinical setting. (IIA26)

10A. What type of cathode and anode are used in polarographic oxygen analyzers?

_____

_____

10B. In what type of fluid are the polarographic cathode and anode immersed?

_____

_____

10C. What happens at the anode and cathode of the polarographic analyzer?

_____

_____

_____

_____

_____

10D. What type of anode and cathode are used in the galvanic oxygen analyzers?

_____

_____

10E. In what type of fluid are the galvanic cathode and anode immersed?

_____

_____

10F. What is the major difference between the polarographic analyzer and the galvanic analyzer?

_____

_____

_____

_____

_____

10G. List three clinical uses for galvanic and polarographic oxygen analyzers.

_____

_____

_____

10H. What situations can affect the readings of a galvanic or polarographic oxygen analyzer?

_____

_____

_____

_____

10I. The electrodes of which type of analyzer last longer and why?

_____

_____

_____

_____

10J. Label the galvanic analyzer shown in Figure 8-12.

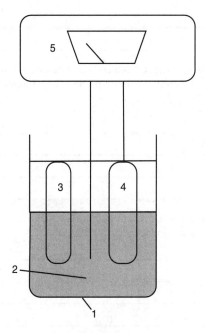

FIGURE 8-12

(1) _____

(2) _____

(3) _____

(4) _____

(5) _____

Think About This:

In what other industries are oxygen analyzers used?

97

11. Describe two techniques for monitoring nitrogen oxides in the clinical setting. (IB9k, IB10k, IIA26)

11A. The administration of what therapeutic gas necessitates monitoring of nitrogen oxides?

_____

_____

11B. What happens to gases sampled by a chemiluminescence monitor?

_____

_____

_____

_____

_____

11C. How is nitrogen dioxide (NO_2) converted to nitric oxide (NO) within the chemiluminescence monitor?

_____

_____

_____

_____

11D. How is the NO_2 concentration determined by the chemiluminescence monitor?

_____

_____

_____

11E. Name four sources of error in a chemiluminescence monitor.

_____

_____

_____

_____

11F. Electrochemical monitoring of nitrogen oxides is based on what principle?

_____

_____

11G. Describe the structure of an electrochemical NO analyzer.

_____

_____

_____

_____

_____

_____

_____

11H. Name two sources of inaccuracy with an electrochemical NO analyzer.

_____

_____

_____

_____

11I. According to the proposed U.S. Food and Drug Administration (FDA) standards for NO and NO_2 monitoring devices, what should the monitoring range, accuracy, and response time be?

_____

_____

_____

_____

_____

_____

11J. Which type of NO monitoring device has a rapid response time, is most accurate, but is also the most expensive?

_____

_____

Think About This:

What role does the measurement of exhaled NO play in airways disease management?

12. Identify the components of a normal capnogram. (IB9c)

12A. Define the term *capnogram*.

_____

12B. What is the fraction of inspired carbon dioxide?

_____

12C. What is the fraction of expired carbon dioxide?

_____

Questions 12D through 12H refer to Figure 8-13.

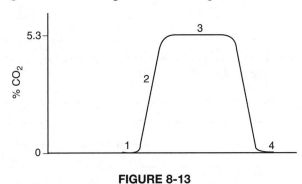

FIGURE 8-13

12D. What is happening during phase 1 of the capnogram?

_____

_____

_____

12E. Why is there an upswing in the capnogram, which is depicted in Figure 8-13 as the line labeled *2*?

_____

_____

_____

_____

12F. What causes phase 3 to have a flat appearance?

_____

_____

12G. At what point on the capnogram is end-tidal partial pressure of carbon dioxide (Pco_2) read?

_____

_____

12H. Why does the capnogram fall to 0 during phase 4?

_____

_____

Think About This:

Are there any other clinical uses for capnography?

13. Assess an abnormal capnogram and suggest possible pathophysiologic processes that could contribute to the contour of the carbon dioxide (CO_2) waveform. (IA7e, IB9c, IB10c, IIIE3d, IIIE4e)

13A. The amount of CO_2 in exhaled air depends on what?

_____

_____

13B. When ventilation and perfusion in the lungs are matched, how much of a difference is there between partial pressure of arterial carbon dioxide ($Paco_2$) and partial pressure of end-tidal CO_2 ($P_{ET}co_2$)?

_____

13C. When ventilation decreases relative to perfusion (V < Q), what happens to $P_{ET}co_2$?

_____

_____

13D. When ventilation increases relative to perfusion (V > Q), what happens to $P_{ET}co_2$?

_____

13E. What are the possible pathophysiologic causes for the capnographic contour shown in Figure 8-14?

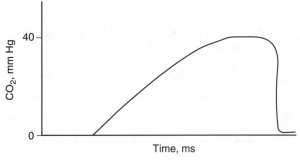

FIGURE 8-14

_____

_____

_____

_____

_____

13F. What is the most likely cause of the capnogram shown in Figure 8-15?

_____

_____

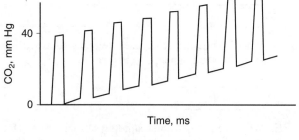

FIGURE 8-15

13G. What is the most likely cause of the capnogram shown in Figure 8-16?

_____

_____

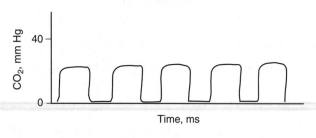

FIGURE 8-16

13H. What are the possible causes of the capnogram shown in Figure 8-17?

_____

_____

_____

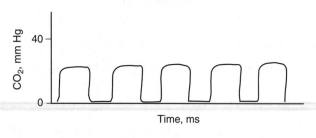

FIGURE 8-17

Think About This:

What would a capnogram look like after a patient had ingested carbonated beverages and was then accidently intubated in the esophagus?

14. Compare closed-circuit and open-circuit indirect calorimeters.

14A. Describe the theory upon which indirect calorimetry is based.

_____

_____

_____

_____

14B. How is oxygen consumption determined by using closed-circuit calorimeters?

_____

_____

_____

_____

14C. How is CO_2 production determined by using closed-circuit calorimeters?

_____

_____

_____

_____

_____

14D. Name three ways that an open-circuit calorimeter measures oxygen consumption.

_____

_____

_____

_____

14E. How do each of these systems operate?

_____

_____

_____

_____

_____

_____

_____

_____

_____

_____

_____

_____

_____

14F. Which type of calorimeter may have problems when used with mechanically ventilated patients? Why?

_____

_____

_____

_____

_____

Think About This:

How can indirect calorimetry be used to manage patients with burns?

15. Calculate energy expenditure by using measurements obtained during indirect calorimetry.

15A. In what two ways can energy expenditure be expressed?

_____

_____

15B. What are the normal values for energy expenditure for a normal, healthy adult?

_____

_____

15C. Calculate the energy expenditure when the oxygen consumption is 250 mL/min and CO_2 production is 200 mL/min.

_____

_____

_____

_____

15D. A 62-year-old male patient with a history of chronic obstructive pulmonary disease (COPD) comes into the emergency department with a report of increasing shortness of breath over the past 3 days. He is hypoxemic and severely hypercapnic and is intubated and placed on mechanical ventilation. Three days later, several attempts to wean him from mechanical ventilation have failed. An indirect calorimetry study was performed and had the following results: oxygen consumption, 230 mL/min; CO_2 production, 220 mL/min. Calculate the patient's energy expenditure.

_____

_____

_____

_____

15E. Calculate the energy expenditure when the oxygen consumption is 270 mL/min and CO_2 production is 235 mL/min.

_____

_____

_____

_____

_____

_____

What effect does infection have on energy expenditure?

16. Explain how indirect calorimetry can be used to determine substrate utilization patterns in healthy individuals and in those with cardiopulmonary dysfunctions.

16A. What are substrate utilization patterns?

_____

_____

_____

_____

_____

16B. What is respiratory quotient (RQ)?

_____

_____

_____

_____

16C. How does indirect calorimetry contribute to substrate utilization patterns?

_____

_____

16D. What is the RQ for the following under normal conditions?

Carbohydrates	
Proteins	
Fat	
Healthy adults	

16E. A mechanically ventilated patient has been unable to complete three weaning attempts. Indirect calorimetry reveals CO_2 production of 173 mL/min and oxygen consumption of 240 mL/min. Calculate the RQ.

_____

_____

16F. Given the circumstances in the previous question, what may be causing this patient's difficulty with weaning?

_____

_____

_____

_____

Think About This:
Does malnutrition have an effect on pulmonary function?

NATIONAL BOARD FOR RESPIRATORY CARE (NBRC)–TYPE QUESTIONS

1. The accuracy of an instrument depends on which of the following?
   1. The standard deviation of repeated measurements
   2. The instrument's linearity and frequency response
   3. The instrument's ability to reproduce a measurement
   4. The instrument's sensitivity to environmental conditions
   A. 1 and 2 only
   B. 1 and 3 only
   C. 2 and 3 only
   D. 2 and 4 only

2. Which is the best method for accurately measuring the thoracic gas volume of a patient with emphysema?
   A. Helium dilution
   B. Nitrogen washout
   C. Pressure plethysmography
   D. Chemiluminescence monitoring

3. After functional residual capacity (FRC) has been measured by using both body plethysmography and nitrogen washout, it is discovered that the FRC measurement from the nitrogen washout test is less than that from the body plethysmographic test. The cause of this discrepancy could be which of the following?
   A. Poor technique
   B. Severe air-trapping
   C. Restrictive lung disease
   D. Directional-valve malfunction

4. The parents of a newborn sent home with an apnea monitor call the respiratory therapist to report that several apnea periods were noted by the monitor's alarm system. The respiratory therapist should check which of the following to ensure that the baby's movement was not the cause of these alarms?
   A. Sensitivity of the monitor
   B. Placement of the electrodes
   C. Amount of electrical current
   D. Frequency of the vibrations

5. Which of the following variables can be measured directly?
   A. Lung compliance
   B. Work of breathing
   C. Airway resistance
   D. Plateau pressure

6. The results of pulmonary function testing show a normal total lung capacity and decreased, but reversible, forced expiratory volume in 1 second (FEV_1) and a forced expiratory flow of 25% to 75% ($FEV_{25\%-75\%}$). The patient is a 22-year-old, nonsmoking male with an intermittent history of "noisy breathing." Which of the following is most likely the cause of his problem?
   A. Asthma
   B. Emphysema
   C. Pulmonary fibrosis
   D. Severe restrictive pulmonary disease

7. What type of device can be incorporated into a ventilator to provide continuous recordings of airway pressure during the breathing cycle?
   A. Variable-capacitance transducer
   B. Inductive plethysmograph
   C. Strain gauge transducer
   D. Aneroid manometer

8. A device that can measure nitric oxide uses which of the following?
   A. Wheatstone bridge
   B. Catalytic converter
   C. Potassium hydroxide
   D. Infrared spectroscope

9. The capnograph in the ventilator circuit is giving an erroneous reading. Which of the following actions is appropriate?
   A. Change the nitrous oxide filter.
   B. Increase the amplifier.
   C. Change the reference cell.
   D. Alter the position of the mirror.

10. A 24-year-old skier with a broken femur has been in the post-anesthesia care unit for 24 hours and is 12 hours post-extubation with no supplemental oxygen. He is awake, alert, and oriented, and he reports shortness of breath. A capnograph shows a decreased partial pressure of end-tidal CO_2 ($P_{ET}CO_2$). Which of the following may explain this patient's current status?
    A. Respiratory center depression
    B. Pulmonary embolism
    C. Muscular paralysis
    D. Alveolar shunt

11. Most calorimeters are unreliable when the oxygen concentration is above 50% to 60% because of which of the following?
    A. Boyle's law
    B. Charles' law
    C. Hamburger effect
    D. Haldane effect

12. What is the expected respiratory quotient of a patient with severe sepsis?
    A. 0.7
    B. 0.8
    C. 1.0
    D. >1.0

13. In Figure 8-18, the amount of pressure required to overcome elastic and frictional forces is represented by which of the following?

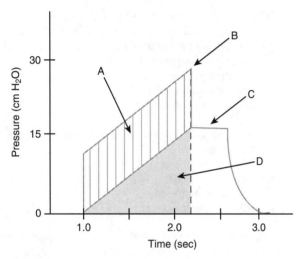

FIGURE 8-18
(From Cairo JM: *Pilbeam's Mechanical ventilation: physiological and clinical applications*, ed 5, St Louis, 2012, Mosby.)

    A. "A"
    B. "B"
    C. "C"
    D. "D"

14. The capnogram seen in Figure 8-19 shows which of the following?

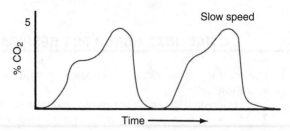

FIGURE 8-19
(From Cairo JM: *Pilbeam's Mechanical ventilation: physiological and clinical applications*, ed 5, St Louis, 2012, Mosby.)

    A. Excessive phase 4
    B. Deep "curare cleft"
    C. Indistinguishable phase 3
    D. Slow cardiac oscillation

15. The arterial-to–end-tidal CO_2 and the arterial-to–maximum expiratory Pco_2 gradients are both elevated and equal to each other. This finding is consistent with which of the following?
    A. Chronic obstructive pulmonary disease
    B. Left-sided heart failure
    C. Esophageal intubation
    D. Pulmonary embolism

9 Assessment of Cardiovascular Function

Upon completion of this chapter, you will be able to:
1. Explain the principles of electrocardiography.
2. Identify the major components of an electrocardiogram.
3. Demonstrate the correct placement of electrodes on a patient to obtain a 12-lead electrocardiogram.
4. Explain the various waves, complexes, and intervals that appear on a normal electrocardiogram.
5. List and describe the most common arrhythmias encountered in clinical electrocardiography.
6. Describe the pressure, volume, and flow events that occur in the heart and major blood vessels during a typical cardiac cycle.
7. Explain the principles of operation of various noninvasive and invasive devices that are routinely used to obtain blood pressure measurements.
8. Describe various invasive and noninvasive methods that are used to measure cardiac output.
9. Interpret hemodynamic measurements that are obtained from patients in a critical care setting.

"The heart has its reasons, which reason does not know." ·
Blaise Pascal

1. Explain the principles of electrocardiography. (IIA19)

1A. What does the electrocardiogram (ECG) represent?

_____

_____

1B. What is meant by a *volume conductor*?

_____

_____

_____

1C. Which electrode is the sensing electrode?

_____

1D. What causes an upward deflection on the ECG's recording paper?

_____

_____

_____

1E. What causes a downward deflection on the ECG's recording paper?

_____

_____

_____

1F. How might heart disease affect an electrocardiographic recording?

_____

_____

_____

Think About This:

Why is there an electrocardiographic tracing during cardiopulmonary resuscitation?

2. Identify the major components of an ECG. (IIA19)

2A. What is the function of the conduction jelly or electrolyte paste used on floating electrodes?

_____

_____

2B. Complete the following table for the augmented leads.

Lead	Positive Electrode	Zero Reference

2C. Name four causes of electrical interference that can occur during electrocardiography.

_____

_____

_____

_____

2D. How far apart are the ruled lines on an ECG paper?

_____

_____

2E. Label the ECG machine in Figure 9-1.

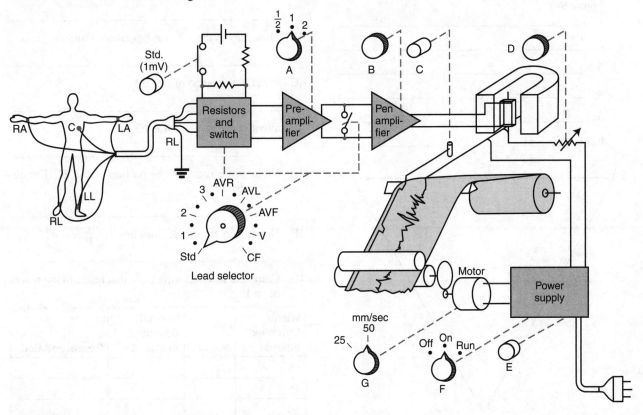

FIGURE 9-1
(Modified from Cromwell L, Weibell FJ, Pfeiffer EA: *Biomedical instrumentation and measurements*, ed 2, Englewood Cliffs, NJ, 1980, Prentice-Hall.)

A. _____   E. _____

B. _____   F. _____

C. _____   G. _____

D. _____

Think About This:
Is it possible to construct a homemade ECG machine?

3. Demonstrate the correct placement of electrodes on a patient to obtain a 12-lead ECG. (IB9a, IIA19)

3A. Circle and number precordial chest lead placement on Figure 9-2.

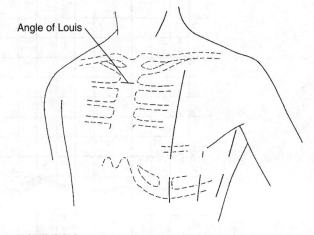

FIGURE 9-2
(From Goldberger AL: *Clinical electrocardiography: a simplified approach*, ed 8, St Louis, 2012, Mosby.)

Chapter **9** **Assessment of Cardiovascular Function**

3B. Identify the components of Einthoven's triangle in Figure 9-3.

1. _____

2. _____

3. _____

4. _____

5. _____

6. _____

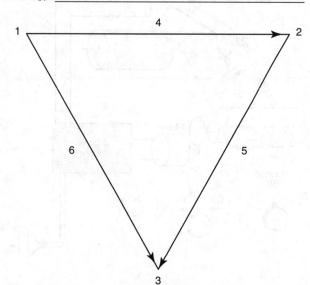

FIGURE 9-3

Think About This:

How would a misplaced lead affect the ECG?

4A. How long is the interval represented by line 1?

_____

4B. How long is the interval represented by line 2?

_____

4C. What is the name of line 3?

_____

4D. What is the name of line 6?

_____

4E. What is the name of the portion of the ECG represented by 13?

_____

4F. How much amplitude does line 16 represent?

_____

4G. Complete the following table that refers to the waves of an ECG.

Wave/ Complex/ Interval	Name	Normal Duration/ Amplitude	Representation
5			
15			
10			
11			
12			
14			

4. Explain the various waves, complexes, and intervals that appear on a normal ECG. (IA8a)

Questions in this section all refer to Figure 9-4.

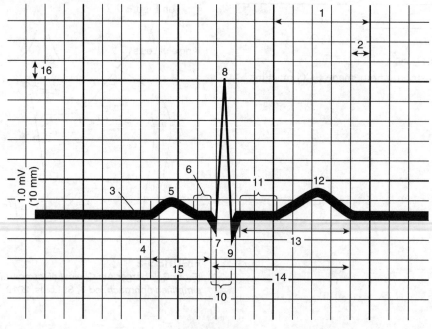

FIGURE 9-4

Think About This:
What is Brugada syndrome?

5. List and describe the most common dysrhythmias encountered in clinical electrocardiography. (IA8a, IB10a)

5A. What is respiratory sinus arrhythmia?

_____

5B. What are the rhythm and rate shown in Figure 9-5? _____

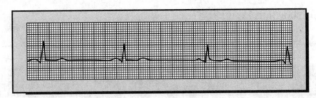

FIGURE 9-5

5C. What type of arrhythmia causes a ventricular rate of >100 bpm with the sinoatrial (SA) node as the source of cardiac excitation?_____

5D. What type of arrhythmia is shown in Figure 9-6? _____

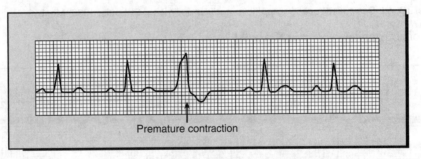

Premature contraction

FIGURE 9-6

5E. What type of arrhythmia is caused by premature atrial depolarizations with prolonged AV conduction time?

_____

5F. Impulses that originate in or near the atrioventricular (AV) node cause what type of a cardiac rhythm?

_____

5G. What type of arrhythmia is shown in Figure 9-7?

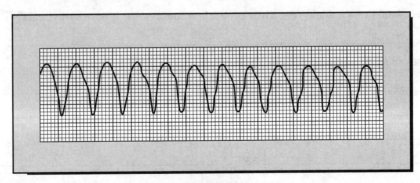

FIGURE 9-7

5H. The presence of a bypass tract in the AV nodes that causes a delta wave following the P wave is known as

_____ .

5I. What arrhythmia causes gross irregularities in both atrial and ventricular depolarizations with an atrial rate between 400 bpm and 700 bpm and a ventricular rate between 120 bpm and 200 bpm?

_____

5J. What type of cardiac arrhythmia causes a "sawtooth" appearance?

_____

5K. What type of arrhythmia is shown in Figure 9-8?

_____

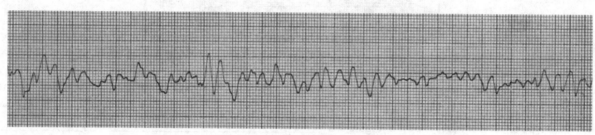

FIGURE 9-8
(From Seidel JC, ed: *Basic electrocardiography: a modular approach*, St Louis, 1986, Mosby.)

5L. What type of arrhythmia is shown in Figure 9-9?

_____

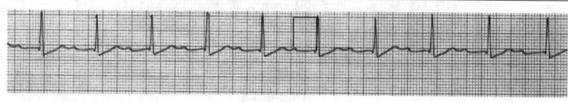

FIGURE 9-9
(From Seidel JC, ed: *Basic electrocardiography: a modular approach*, St Louis, 1986, Mosby.)

5M. Describe the difference between a Mobitz type I block and a Mobitz type II block.

_____

_____

_____

5N. A complete dissociation of atrial and ventricular conduction causes what type of arrhythmia?

_____

5O. Name five causes of right bundle branch blocks.

_____

_____

_____

_____

_____

5P. Name two causes of left bundle branch blocks.

_____

_____

Think About This:

What types of arrhythmias can tracheobronchial suctioning cause?

6. Describe the pressure, volume, and flow events that occur in the heart and major blood vessels during a typical cardiac cycle.

6A. What are the two main parts of the cardiac cycle?

_____

_____

6B. What electrocardiographic waveform corresponds with isovolumetric contraction?

_____

6C. Why does the volume in the ventricles remain constant during isovolumetric contraction of the heart?

_____

_____

6D. How much pressure is generated in the left and right ventricles during isovolumetric contraction?

_____

6E. What opens the semilunar valves of the heart?

_____

_____

6F. What are the peak systolic pressures in the left and right ventricles?

_____

Questions 6G through 6K refer to Figure 9-10.

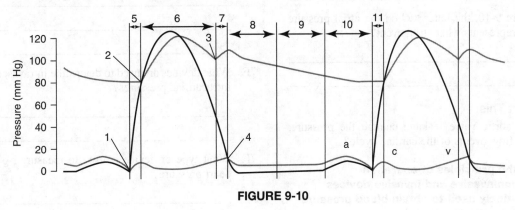

FIGURE 9-10

6G. At what points on Figure 9-10 do the following events occur?

Mitral valve closes _____   Aortic valve opens _____

Aortic valve closes _____   Mitral valve opens _____

6H. Identify the cardiac flow events that are indicated by the following points on Figure 9-10.

Point 5 _____

_____

Point 6 _____

_____

Point 7 _____

_____

Point 8 _____

_____

Point 9 _____

_____

Point 10 _____

_____

Point 11 _____

_____

6I. In Figure 9-10, the letter "a" on the atrial pressure tracing represents what atrial event?

_____

_____

6J. In Figure 9-10, the letter "c" on the atrial pressure tracing represents what atrial event?

_____

_____

6K. In Figure 9-10, the letter "v" on the atrial pressure tracing represents what atrial event?

_____

_____

Think About This:

How would aortic valve leakage change the pressure, volume, and flow events of the cardiac cycle?

7. Explain the principles of operation of various noninvasive and invasive devices that are routinely used to obtain blood pressure measurements. (IIA20a, IIA20b)

7A. How does a sphygmomanometer measure blood pressure?

_____

_____

_____

_____

_____

_____

_____

_____

_____

_____

_____

7B. Why does the tapping sound disappear when measuring noninvasive blood pressure?

_____

_____

7C. How are pressure pulsations detected with an automated blood pressure system?

_____

_____

_____

7D. What are the errors most commonly encountered while determining arterial blood pressure with either a manual or an automated blood pressure monitoring system?

_____

_____

_____

_____

7E. What devices are used to determine intravascular and intracardiac pressures?

_____

_____

7F. What type of device is used to measure right-sided heart pressure?

_____

_____

7G. Explain the purpose of each lumen of a four-lumen thermodilution catheter.

_____

_____

_____

_____

_____

_____

_____

_____

_____

7H. How are aortic pressure, left ventricular pressure, and left atrium pressure measured?

_____

_____

_____

_____

7I. What is the transseptal approach to left-sided heart catheterization?

_____

_____

_____

_____

7J. Name the three types of pressure transducers.

_____

_____

_____

_____

7K. Which pressure transducers are the most frequently used?

_____

_____

Think About This:

Why must a left-sided heart catheterization be performed in the cardiac catheterization lab, whereas right-sided heart catheterization can be performed at the bedside?

8. Describe various methods that are used to measure cardiac output. (IB9m)

8A. What information is necessary to use Fick's direct method of calculating cardiac output?

_____

_____

_____

_____

8B. What is the formula for Fick's direct method?

_____

8C. How is cardiac output measured with use of the indicator dilution method?

_____

_____

_____

_____

_____

_____

_____

_____

8D. How is cardiac output measured with use of the thermodilution technique?

_____

_____

_____

_____

_____

_____

_____

8E. How is impedance plethysmography used to determine cardiac output?

_____

_____

_____

_____

_____

8F. How is impedance cardiography used to measure cardiac output?

_____

_____

_____

_____

8G. How is transesophageal Doppler used to measure cardiac output?

_____

_____

_____

_____

8H. What is the difference between the Fick's direct and the Fick's indirect method of calculating cardiac output?

_____

_____

_____

_____

Think About This:

Does respiratory variation in pulmonary blood flow cause changes in cardiac output measurements?

9. Interpret hemodynamic measurements that are obtained from patients in a critical care setting. (IA8b, IB10m, IIIE4c)

9A. How can tachycardia lead to decreased cardiac output?

_____

_____

9B. What factors are the focus of a hemodynamic profile?

_____

_____

9C. What measurements are used to estimate right ventricular end-diastolic pressure and left ventricular end-diastolic pressure?

_____

_____

9D. What are two reasons for a reduction in cardiac output?

_____

_____

9E. Complete the following table with the equations and normal ranges for each hemodynamic measurement.

Hemodynamic Measurement	Formula	Normal Range
Cardiac output (Q)		
Cardiac index (CI)		
Stroke index (SI)		

Systemic vascular resistance (SVR)		
Pulmonary vascular resistance (PVR)		
Left ventricular *stroke work* (LSW)		
Right ventricular stroke work (RSW)		
Left ventricular *stroke work index* (LSWI)		
Right ventricular stroke work index (RSWI)		

9F. A 55-year-old female patient is admitted to the emergency department with ischemic heart disease requiring three coronary artery bypass grafts. After surgery, the patient is maintained on mechanical ventilation. She has an intraaortic balloon pump and a pulmonary artery catheter in place. Use the following data to calculate the patient's cardiac index, stroke index, LSWI, RSWI, SVR, and PVR.

Body surface area = 1.7 m^2 $\dot{Q}$ = 4.0 L/min

Mean arterial pressure = 68 mm Hg

Mean pulmonary artery pressure = 36 mm Hg
Pulmonary capillary wedge pressure = 14 mm Hg
Central venous pressure = 18 mm Hg

Heart rate = 98 bpm

_____

_____

_____

_____

_____

_____

_____

_____

_____

_____

_____

Think About This:

Are hemodynamic profiles appropriate for all mechanically ventilated patients?

NATIONAL BOARD FOR RESPIRATORY CARE (NBRC)–TYPE QUESTIONS

1. β-Adrenergic blocking agents, such as propranolol, can cause which of the following?
   A. Sinoatrial (SA) block
   B. Sinus tachycardia
   C. Sinus bradycardia
   D. Premature atrial beats

2. Failure of the SA node to depolarize or failure of the atrioventricular (AV) node to conduct impulses will result in which of the following cardiac arrhythmias?
   A. Atrial fibrillation
   B. Junctional escape rhythm
   C. Premature ventricular beats
   D. Paroxysmal atrial tachycardia

3. The heart block that causes "dropped" beats and that is often the result of increased parasympathetic tone is which of the following?
   A. SA block
   B. Mobitz type I block
   C. First-degree AV block
   D. Left bundle branch block

4. "Pressure rises in the ventricles, but no blood is ejected" is the definition of which of the following?
   A. Ventricular systole
   B. Ventricular diastole
   C. Isovolumetric relaxation
   D. Isovolumetric contraction

5. The right ventricle peak systolic pressure is how many mm Hg?
   A. 15
   B. 25
   C. 80
   D. 120

6. Closure of the semilunar valves and opening of the AV valves is associated with which heart sound?
   A. S1
   B. S2
   C. S3
   D. S4

7. The respiratory therapist is unable to "wedge" the pulmonary artery catheter 24 hours after insertion. The problem is most likely caused by which of the following?
   A. Pneumothorax
   B. Balloon rupture
   C. Catheter knotting
   D. Pulmonary artery rupture

8. Use Fick's direct method to calculate cardiac output for a patient with the following hemodynamic values.

Partial pressure of arterial oxygen (PaO_2) = 80 mm Hg	Hemoximetry oxygen saturation (SaO_2) = 90%	Hemoglobin = 14 g/dL
Partial pressure of oxygen in mixed venous blood ($P_{\bar{v}}O_2$) = 35 mm Hg	Saturation of oxygen in mixed venous blood ($S_{\bar{v}}O_2$) = 65%	P_{bar} = 760 mm Hg
	Oxygen consumption ($\dot{V}O_2$) = 210 mL/min	

   A. 3.5 L/min
   B. 4.36 L/min
   C. 5.83 L/min
   D. 6.15 L/min

9. Calculate cardiac index when cardiac output = 5.0 L/min and body surface area = 2.9 m².
   A. 1.72 L/min/m²
   B. 1.67 L/min/m²
   C. 2.10 L/min/m²
   D. 12.5 L/min/m²

10. Calculation of systemic vascular resistance is 1700 dyne sec/cm⁻⁵. Which of the following is consistent with this value?
   A. Elevated left ventricular afterload
   B. Elevated right ventricular afterload
   C. Decreased left ventricular preload
   D. Decreased right ventricular preload

10

Blood Gas Monitoring

Upon completion of this chapter, you will be able to:
1. Describe how to perform and evaluate the modified Allen's test.
2. Identify various sites used to obtain samples for blood gas analysis.
3. Label the components of a modern, in vitro blood gas analyzer.
4. Compare the operational principles of the pH, partial pressure of carbon dioxide (PCO_2), and partial pressure of oxygen (PO_2) electrodes.
5. Apply values for PO_2 at which 50% saturation of hemoglobin (P_{50}) occurs, as well as for bicarbonate, buffer base, and base excess, in the interpretation of arterial blood gases (ABGs).
6. Explain the operational principle of carbon monoxide (CO) oximetry.
7. Name the components of a quality assurance program for blood gas analysis.
8. Compare the effects of hyperthermia and hypothermia on ABGs.
9. Describe physiologic and technical factors that can affect pulse oximeter readings.
10. Identify various factors that can influence transcutaneous PO_2 and PCO_2 measurements.
11. State the criteria for identifying four types of acid-base disorders.

"You know you're old if they have discontinued your blood type."
Phyllis Diller

ACHIEVING THE OBJECTIVES

1. Describe how to perform and evaluate the modified Allen's test. (IB9f)

1A. When should the modified Allen's test be used?

_____

_____

1B. Why does a patient need to clench her fist during the Allen's test?

_____

_____

1C. Identify the two blood vessels depicted in Figure 10-1.

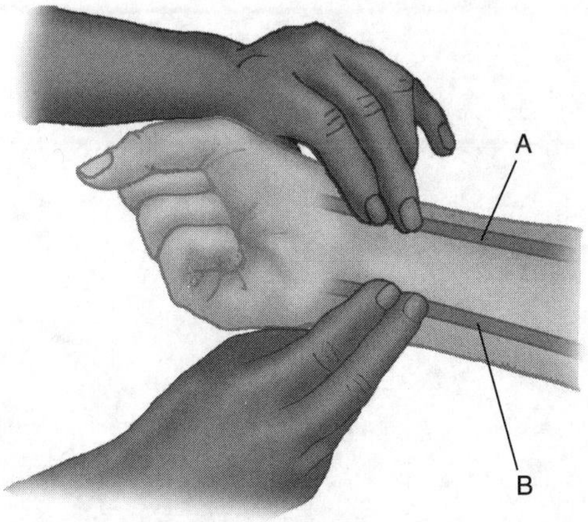

FIGURE 10-1
(From Kacmarek RM, Stoller JK, Heuer AJ: *Egan's fundamentals of respiratory care*, ed 10, St Louis, 2013, Mosby.)

_____

_____

1D. What is the purpose of applying pressure to both blood vessels shown in Figure 10-1?

_____

_____

1E. How should the hand appear when the patient releases his fist while the vessels are occluded?

_____

_____

1F. Which blood vessel is released first?

_____

1G. How do you assess a negative result for the Allen's test?

_____

_____

_____

1H. How do you assess a positive result for the Allen's test?

_____

_____

_____

1I. What should you do if the result of the Allen's test is negative? What should you do if the result of the Allen's test is positive?

_____

_____

_____

_____

_____

Think About This:
Can an Allen's test be performed on an unconscious patient?

2. Identify various sites used to obtain samples for blood gas analysis. (IB9f)

2A. Identify and label the four most common percutaneous sampling sites in Figure 10-2.

_____

_____

_____

_____

2B. Through what type of catheter are mixed venous blood samples drawn?

_____

_____

2C. Capillary blood samples can be drawn from what site?

_____

_____

Think About This:

Why does the bevel of the needle need to be facing up when you are drawing an arterial blood gas sample?

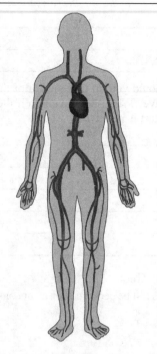

FIGURE 10-2
(From Kacmarek RM, Stoller JK, Heuer AJ: *Egan's fundamentals of respiratory care*, ed 10, St Louis, 2013, Mosby.)

3. Label the components of a modern, in vitro blood gas analyzer. (IIA9)

3A. Label the pH electrode shown in Figure 10-3.

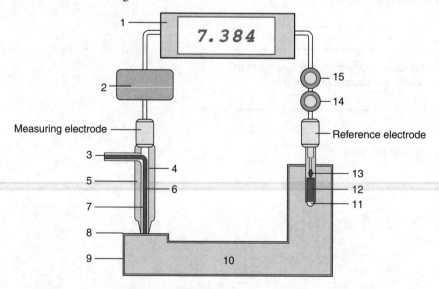

FIGURE 10-3

1. _____	2. _____	3. _____
4. _____	5. _____	6. _____
7. _____	8. _____	9. _____
10. _____	11. _____	12. _____
13. _____	14. _____	15. _____

3B. Label the Stow-Severinghaus electrode shown in Figure 10-4.

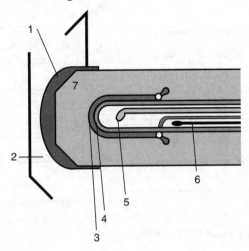

FIGURE 10-4
(Redrawn from Shapiro BA, Peruzzi WT, Templin R: *Clinical application of blood gases*, ed 5, St Louis, 1994, Mosby.)

1. _____	2. _____	3. _____
4. _____	5. _____	6. _____
7. _____		

3C. Label the Clark electrode shown in Figure 10-5.

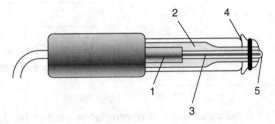

FIGURE 10-5
(From Shapiro BA, Peruzzi WT, Templin R: *Clinical application of blood gases*, ed 5, St Louis, 1994, Mosby.)

| 1. _____ | 2. _____ | 3. _____ |
| 4. _____ | 5. _____ | |

Think About This:
What other uses do pH, partial pressure of carbon dioxide (PCO_2), and partial pressure of oxygen (PO_2) electrodes have?

4. **Compare the operational principles of the pH, PCO$_2$, and PO$_2$ electrodes. (IIA9)**

4A. Which electrode has a silver anode and a platinum cathode?

_____

_____

4B. Which electrode incorporates a permeable silicone elastic membrane?

_____

_____

4C. Which electrode has a calomel reference half-cell and a silver–silver chloride electrode?

_____

_____

4D. The pH electrode uses what two immersion solutions?

_____

_____

4E. What immersion solution does the PCO$_2$ electrode use?

_____

4F. What immersion solution does the PO$_2$ electrode use?

_____

4G. What type of measurement technique is used in the pH electrode?

_____

_____

_____

_____

_____

4H. What type of measurement technique does the PCO$_2$ electrode use?

_____

_____

_____

_____

_____

4I. The PO$_2$ electrode uses what type of measurement technique?

_____

_____

_____

_____

4J. What equation represents what occurs within the pH electrode?

_____

_____

4K. The chemical reaction that occurs in the immersion solution of the PCO$_2$ electrode is

_____ ,

_____ .

4L. How is pH related to the PCO$_2$?

_____

_____

_____

Think About This:

What other types of chemical electrodes exist?

5. **Apply values for PO$_2$ at which 50% saturation of hemoglobin occurs (P$_{50}$), as well as for bicarbonate, buffer base, and base excess, in the interpretation of arterial blood gases (ABGs). (IIIE4a; IB10j; IB10f)**

5A. Take the following factors into account.

pH 7.22	Partial pressure of arterial carbon dioxide (PaCO$_2$) 55 mm Hg	Bicarbonate (HCO$_3^-$) 25 mEq/L	Partial pressure of arterial oxygen (PaO$_2$) 60 mm Hg	Hemoximetry oxygen saturation (SaO$_2$) 88%
Fractional inspired oxygen (F$_I$O$_2$) nasal cannula (NC) 3 L/min	Age 45			

Offer your interpretation of these data:

_____

_____

5B. Take the following factors into account.

pH 7.32	PaCO$_2$ 32 mm Hg	HCO$_3$$^-$ 18 mEq/L	PaO$_2$ 101 mm Hg	SaO$_2$ 97%
F$_I$O$_2$ room air	Age 58			

Offer your interpretation of these data:

_____

5C. Take the following factors into account.

pH 7.43	PaCO$_2$ 48 mm Hg	HCO$_3$$^-$ 36 mEq/L	PaO$_2$ 91 mm Hg	SaO$_2$ 97%
F$_I$O$_2$ NC 3 L/min	Age 66			

Offer your interpretation of these data:

_____

5D. Take the following factors into account.

pH 7.48	PaCO$_2$ 22 mm Hg	HCO$_3$$^-$ 16 mEq/L	PaO$_2$ 96 mm Hg	SaO$_2$ 98%
F$_I$O$_2$ room air	Age 18			

Offer your interpretation of these data:

_____

Use Figure 10-6 to complete questions 5E through 5G.

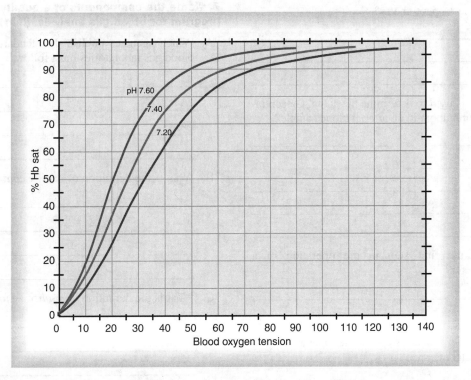

FIGURE 10-6
(From Kacmarek RM, Stoller JK, Heuer AJ: *Egan's fundamentals of respiratory care*, ed 10, St Louis, 2013, Mosby.)

5E. What is the P_{50} for a pH of 7.60?

_____

5F. What is the P_{50} for a pH of 7.40?

_____

5G. What is the P_{50} for a pH of 7.20?

_____

5H. A low P_{50} represents what type of change in the oxy-hemoglobin dissociation curve?

_____

5I. A high P_{50} represents what type of change in the oxyhemoglobin dissociation curve?

_____
_____

Think About This:

Are the ABGs of other animals similar to those of humans?

6. Explain the operational principle of carbon monoxide (CO) oximetry. (IIA26)

6A. What values does an in vitro CO-oximeter measure?

_____
_____

6B. What is spectrophotometry?

_____
_____
_____

6C. What law is used to determine the actual concentration of hemoglobin in an arterial blood sample?

_____
_____
_____
_____

6D. What is the first step in the operation of a CO-oximeter?

_____
_____

6E. What is the second step in the operation of a CO-oximeter?

_____
_____

6F. How is light transmission measured by means of the CO-oximeter?

_____
_____
_____
_____
_____
_____

6G. What factors interfere with CO-oximetry measurements?

_____
_____
_____
_____
_____
_____
_____

Think About This:

What advantage does fetal hemoglobin provide by causing a left shift in the oxygen dissociation curve?

7. Name the components of a quality assurance program for blood gas analysis. (IIC1)

7A. Which agencies publish the standards that clinical blood gas laboratories must follow?

_____
_____
_____

7B. What is the definition of *quality control*?

_____
_____
_____
_____

7C. What is the definition of *quality assurance*?

_____
_____
_____

7D. What are the components of a quality assurance program for blood gas analysis?

_____

_____

_____

_____

_____

7E. How is blood gas analyzer proficiency testing accomplished?

_____

_____

_____

_____

_____

_____

7F. What are the generally acceptable limits for pH, PCO_2, and PO_2 in proficiency testing?

_____

_____

_____

_____

Think About This:

What steps need to be taken to obtain a Clinical Laboratory Improvement Amendments certification for a blood gas lab?

8. Compare the effect of hyperthermia and hypothermia on ABGs. (IIA9)

8A. What effect does temperature have on the PaO_2?

_____

_____

8B. For every degree Celsius, how much will the $PaCO_2$ change?

_____

8C. For every degree Celsius, how much will the pH change?

_____

8D. What happens to the oxyhemoglobin dissociation curve when the patient is hypothermic?

_____

_____

_____

_____

8E. What happens to the oxyhemoglobin dissociation curve when the patient is hyperthermic?

_____

_____

_____

_____

Think About This:

Why is there such a controversy over temperature correction for ABG parameters?

9. Describe physiologic and technical factors that can affect pulse oximeter readings. (IB9c; IB10c; IIA22)

9A. Why do low perfusion states cause intermittent or absent saturations when measured by pulse oximetry?

_____

_____

9B. Name three physiologic causes and one technical cause of low perfusion states.

_____

_____

_____

_____

9C. How can the problem of low perfusion states be prevented when pulse oximetry is used?

_____

_____

9D. How do high levels of carboxyhemoglobin alter pulse oximetry oxygen saturation (SpO_2) measurements?

_____

_____

_____

_____

9E. What type of hemoglobin absorbs both red and infrared light?

_____

9F. How will this type of hemoglobin (from question 9E) affect the pulse oximeter reading?

_____

_____

_____

_____

9G. What can cause the production of the hemoglobin discussed in questions 9E and 9F?

_____

_____

9H. During cardiac catheterizations, what might cause a false drop in the patient's SpO_2?

_____

_____

_____

9I. How do dark nail polishes affect SpO_2 readings?

_____

_____

_____

_____

9J. What types of light sources might adversely affect heart rate and SpO_2 readings?

_____

_____

9K. How do pulse oximeters compensate for ambient light interference?

_____

_____

_____

_____

Think About This:

What role does pulse oximetry play in the diagnosis of sleep apnea?

10. Identify various factors that can influence transcutaneous PO_2 and PCO_2 measurements. (IB9b; IB10b; IIA22; IIC7; IIIE3a)

10A. How could a heater failure of the transcutaneous PO_2 electrode affect its ability to measure?

_____

_____

_____

_____

10B. How are transcutaneous PO_2 ($PtCO_2$) measurements influenced by peripheral perfusion?

_____

_____

_____

10C. Which pathologic states can lead to erroneous $PtCO_2$ measurements in a patient?

_____

_____

_____

_____

10D. What effect does a decreasing cardiac index have on the accuracy of $PtCO_2$ measurements?

_____

_____

_____

_____

10E. Why does heating a carbon dioxide electrode cause a slightly higher reading of the $PtCO_2$ than the $PaCO_2$?

_____

_____

10F. Why should the site for the electrode placement be prepped by cleansing and (if necessary) shaving?

_____

_____

10G. What potential adverse effect can the heat at the electrode site cause?

_____

_____

_____

_____

10H. Why should electrodes be cleaned periodically?

_____

_____

10I. Why should the electrolyte and the sensor's membranes be checked regularly?

_____

_____

Think About This:
Are there other uses for transcutaneous electrodes?

11. State the criteria for identifying four types of acid-base disorders. (IB10f; IB10j; IIIE4a)

11A. What are the criteria for metabolic acidosis?

Type of Metabolic Acidosis	pH	PCO$_2$	HCO$_3^-$
Acute			
Partly compensated			
Compensated			

11B. What are the criteria for respiratory acidosis?

Type of Respiratory Acidosis	pH	PCO$_2$	HCO$_3^-$
Acute			
Partly compensated			
Compensated			

11C. What are the criteria for metabolic alkalosis?

Type of Metabolic Alkalosis	pH	PCO$_2$	HCO$_3^-$
Acute			
Partly compensated			
Compensated			

11D. What are the criteria for respiratory alkalosis?

Type of Respiratory Alkalosis	pH	PCO$_2$	HCO$_3^-$
Acute			
Partly compensated			
Compensated			

Interpret the following results in terms of acid-base balance.

	pH	PCO$_2$	HCO$_3^-$	Interpretation
11E.	7.28	60	24	
11F.	7.38	96	32	
11G.	7.52	28	20	
11H.	7.44	28	19	
11I.	7.46	34	23	
11J.	7.28	80	37	
11K.	7.59	49	48	
11L.	7.34	38	21	
11M.	7.44	48	33	
11N.	7.36	30	15	
11O.	7.51	39	31	
11P.	7.34	34	18	

Think About This:

What are the normal and abnormal acid-base values for dogs, cats, and other nonhuman animals?

NATIONAL BOARD FOR RESPIRATORY CARE (NBRC)–TYPE QUESTIONS

1. What is the correct sequence of events when one is obtaining arterial blood from the radial artery of a patient?
   1. Perform a modified Allen's test.
   2. Remove any air bubbles from the sample.
   3. Apply direct pressure to the puncture site.
   4. Clean the puncture site with a suitable antiseptic solution.
   5. Use a 23-gauge needle and a plastic syringe containing an anticoagulant.
   A. 1, 4, 3, 5, 2
   B. 4, 1, 5, 2, 3
   C. 1, 4, 5, 3, 2

2. What is the correct order of steps to perform a modified Allen's test?
   1. Pressure is applied to both the radial and ulnar arteries.
   2. The fist is opened, but the fingers are not fully extended.
   3. Pressure on the ulnar artery is removed.
   4. The hand is clenched into a tight fist.
   5. The palm and fingers are blanched.
   A. 4, 1, 2, 5, 3
   B. 4, 5, 1, 3, 2
   C. 1, 4, 3, 2, 5
   D. 4, 2, 1, 3, 5

3. The reference half-cell of a pH analyzer is composed of which of the following?
   A. Silver anode
   B. Platinum cathode
   C. Silver–silver chloride
   D. Mercury–mercurous chloride

4. In a partial pressure of carbon dioxide (PCO_2) electrode, carbon dioxide
   1. Reacts with potassium chloride.
   2. Reacts with water to form carbonic acid.
   3. Diffuses through a silicon elastic membrane.
   4. Diffuses through a semipermeable plastic membrane.
   A. 2 and 3 only
   B. 1 and 3 only
   C. 1 and 4 only
   D. 2 and 4 only

5. Erroneous PCO_2 measurements may be caused by which of the following?
   1. A cracked electrode
   2. Wearing out of the silver anode

3. Increased temperature of the patient
4. Dehydration of bicarbonate solution
   A. 1 and 2 only
   B. 1 and 4 only
   C. 2 and 3 only
   D. 3 and 4 only

6. Which of the following variables is measured directly?
   A. Partial pressure of oxygen at which hemoglobin is 50% saturated (P_{50})
   B. Partial pressure of arterial oxygen (PaO_2)
   C. HCO_3^-
   D. Hemoximetry oxygen saturation (SaO_2)

7. Which of the following would create the highest P_{50}?
   A. pH = 7.40
   B. pH = 7.50
   C. PCO_2 = 40 mm Hg
   D. PCO_2 = 60 mm Hg

8. What type of calibration should be performed after an electrode is changed?
   A. Quality control
   B. Three-point
   C. Two-point
   D. One-point

9. Quality control includes which of the following?
   1. Analyzing unknown samples and submitting to the sponsoring organization
   2. Comparing control sample measurements against defined limits
   3. Addressing problems through corrective actions
   4. Identifying problems
   A. 1 and 2 only
   B. 3 and 4 only
   C. 2, 3, and 4 only
   D. 1, 2, 3, and 4

10. What are the two bases of operation for pulse oximetry?
    1. Optical plethysmography
    2. Impedance plethysmography
    3. Spectrophotometry
    4. Potentiometry
    A. 1 and 3 only
    B. 2 and 4 only
    C. 1 and 4 only
    D. 2 and 3 only

127

11. A patient is being treated with dapsone, an antibiotic, for *Pneumocystis carinii*. Which of the following ways of measuring oxygen saturation would be most appropriate?
   A. In vivo blood gas monitoring
   B. In vitro blood gas monitoring
   C. Pulse oximetry
   D. Carbon monoxide (CO) oximetry

12. A patient undergoing continuous pulse oximetry is receiving supplemental oxygen. The pulse oximetry oxygen saturation (SpO_2) has been 93% ± 2 for the past 12 hours. The pulse oximeter suddenly sounds an alarm and reads 78%. A rapid assessment reveals cyanosis and shortness of breath. What should your immediate action be?
   A. Take an arterial blood gas measurement without delay.
   B. Recalibrate the pulse oximeter.
   C. Change the pulse oximeter probe.
   D. Decrease the supplemental oxygen.

13. Which of the following cause erroneous transcutaneous partial pressure of oxygen ($PtCO_2$) readings?
   1. Hypovolemia
   2. Hypothermia
   3. Septic shock
   4. Asthma
      A. 1 and 3 only
      B. 1 and 4 only
      C. 1, 2, and 3 only
      D. 2, 3, and 4 only

14. The following arterial blood gas results — pH = 7.37; PCO_2 = 55 mm Hg; PO_2 = 53 mm Hg; SaO_2 = 88%; HCO_3^- = 31 mEq/L can be interpreted as:
   A. Compensated metabolic alkalosis with mild hypoxemia.
   B. Compensated respiratory acidosis with moderate hypoxemia.
   C. Partially compensated respiratory acidosis with mild hypoxemia.
   D. Partially compensated respiratory acidosis with severe hypoxemia.

15. Analyze the following acid-base balance: pH = 7.35; PCO_2 = 22 mm Hg; HCO_3^- = 12 mEq/L. What would be your interpretation of these data?
   A. Combined alkalemia
   B. Combined acidemia
   C. Compensated respiratory alkalemia
   D. Compensated metabolic acidosis

Sleep Diagnostics

Upon completion of this chapter, you will be able to:
1. Describe the various stages of sleep in adults and children.
2. Discuss the physiologic effects of sleep on cardiopulmonary function in healthy individuals.
3. List the measurements most commonly recorded during polysomnography.
4. Summarize the clinical and laboratory criteria used to diagnose obstructive, central, and mixed apnea.
5. Describe various strategies that can be used to monitor arterial oxygen saturation, nasal–oral airflow, and respiratory effort of patients with obstructive sleep apnea syndrome.
6. Explain the physiologic consequences of obstructive sleep apnea.
7. Name several common diseases associated with central sleep apnea.

"People need dreams; there's as much nourishment in 'em as food."
Dorothy Gilman

1. Describe the various stages of sleep in adults and children. (IA10)

1A. What are the two distinct states of sleep?

    1. _____

    2. _____

1B. What are the electrographic and behavioral differences between these two states of sleep for individuals 12 months of age and older?

_____

_____

_____

_____

_____

1C. Which sleep stage is known as *quiet sleep*?

_____

1D. Which waveforms are present during wakefulness and during the onset of quiet sleep?

_____

1E. Describe the electroencephalographic and electro-oculographic findings during stage 1 of quiet sleep.

_____

_____

_____

_____

_____

1F. How is the transition to stage 2 of quiet sleep identified?

_____

_____

_____

_____

_____

1G. What does the electro-oculogram show during stage 2?

_____

1H. What enables you to distinguish stage 3 from the other stages?

_____

_____

1I. How are stages 3 and 4 differentiated in the R&K Scoring System?

_____

_____

_____

_____

_____

_____

1J. How long does non–rapid eye movement (non-REM) sleep usually last?

_____

1K. What stage of sleep is known as *slow-wave sleep*?

_____

1L. What type of waveform is present during rapid eye movement (REM) sleep?

_____

_____

_____

1M. Dreams that are remembered occur during which state of sleep?

_____

1N. What is the sleep-stage distribution in normal, healthy adults?

_____

_____

_____

1O. How long does REM sleep usually last during a typical 8-hour period of sleep in a healthy adult?

_____

Think About This:

Why do infants spend most of their sleep in REM?

2. Discuss the physiologic effects of sleep on cardiopulmonary function in healthy individuals.

2A. During which stages of sleep is a person predisposed to apneic periods?

_____

_____

_____

_____

_____

_____

_____

2B. How does minute ventilation change during non-REM slow-wave sleep?

_____

_____

2C. What happens to the partial pressure of arterial oxygen (PaO_2) and the partial pressure of arterial carbon dioxide ($PaCO_2$) during non-REM slow-wave sleep?

_____

_____

2D. During which sleep stage is there an increase in upper airway resistance?

_____

2E. What effect does sleep have on heart rate and blood pressure?

_____

_____

_____

_____

_____

_____

_____

_____

2F. During which stage of sleep is cardiac output reduction pronounced?

_____

_____

2G. What effect does sleep have on blood vessels?

_____

_____

_____

Think About This:

Can sleep disturbances cause permanent cardiovascular problems?

3. List the measurements most commonly recorded during polysomnography. (IB9a, IB9c, IC13)

3A. How is cardiac function measured during polysomnography? _____

3B. How are the stages of sleep identified?

_____

3C. What four physiologic parameters of breathing are measured?

1. _____

2. _____

3. _____

4. _____

3D. What are the most common ways of measuring the parameters answered in question 3C?

_____

_____

_____

_____

_____

_____

_____

3E. How are arousal responses and movements monitored during polysomnography?

_____

_____

_____

3F. What measurement is used to assess eye movement during polysomnography?

_____

_____

_____

_____

Think About This:

Why is continuous video monitoring important during polysomnography?

4. Summarize the clinical and laboratory criteria used to diagnose obstructive, central, and mixed apnea. (IA10, IC13)

4A. What does a patient with obstructive sleep apnea (OSA) typically report?

_____

_____

_____

4B. What are the criteria for the diagnosis of OSA?

_____

_____

_____

_____

_____

_____

4C. How can OSA be differentiated from central sleep apnea (CSA)?

_____

_____

_____

4D. How can mixed sleep apnea be differentiated from OSA and CSA?

_____

_____

4E. Identify the type of sleep apnea shown in Figure 11-1.

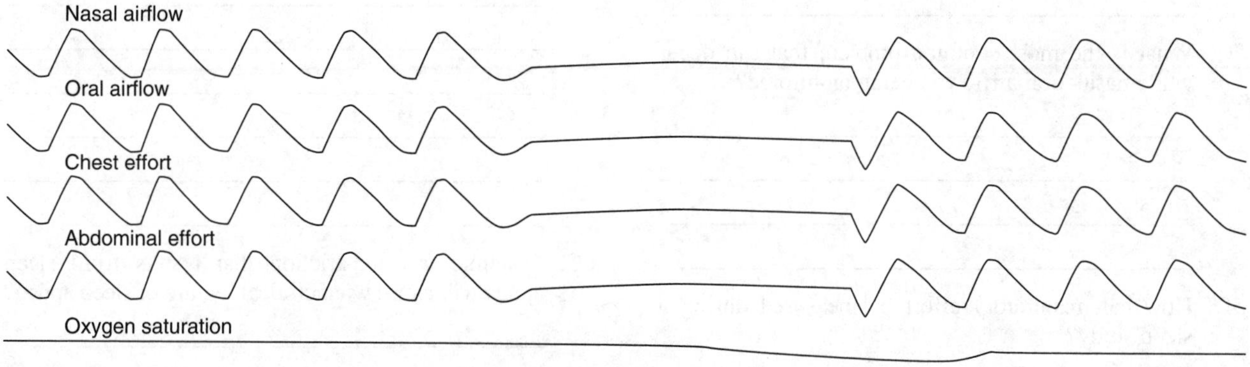

_____

FIGURE 11-1
(Redrawn from Sheldon SH, Spire JP, Levy HB: *Pediatric sleep medicine,* Philadelphia, 1992, WB Saunders.)

4F. What type of individual has the greatest risk for developing OSA?

_____

_____

4G. What other factors increase an individual's risk for OSA?

_____

_____

4H. What factors may augment the symptoms of patients with mild OSA?

_____

_____

Think About This:

How is neonatal apnea diagnosed?

5. **Describe various strategies that can be used to monitor arterial oxygen saturation, nasal–oral airflow, and the respiratory effort of patients with OSA syndrome. (IB9c, IC8, IC13, IIA17)**

5A. How is oxygen saturation monitored during polysomnography?

_____

_____

5B. How is nasal–oral airflow monitored during a sleep study?

_____

_____

_____

5C. What is the most common problem that can occur while nasal–oral airflow is being monitored?

_____

_____

_____

5D. How can respiratory effort be measured during a sleep study?

_____

_____

_____

_____

_____

5E. What equipment can be used to monitor respiratory effort?

_____

_____

_____

_____

_____

Think About This:

What role do home sleep studies play in the diagnosis of sleep apnea?

6. **Explain the physiologic consequences of OSA.**

6A. What physiologic consequence of sleep apnea causes "unexplained" nocturnal death?

_____

_____

_____

6B. How do pulmonary hypertension and right-sided heart failure develop as a result of sleep apnea?

_____

_____

_____

_____

6C. Systemic vasoconstriction that results from sleep apnea will cause what clinical feature of sleep apnea?

_____

6D. What are the physiologic causes of excessive daytime sleepiness, personality changes, intellectual deterioration, and behavioral disorders commonly observed in patients with sleep apnea?

_____

_____

_____

_____

_____

6E. Restless sleep in sleep apnea is a consequence of what physiologic process?

_____

Think About This:

What effect does OSA have on diabetes?

7. Name several diseases commonly associated with CSA.

7A. What three mechanisms have been suggested as accountable for the cessation of respiratory drive associated with CSA?

1. _____

2. _____

3. _____

7B. Name three kinds of diseases that are associated with CSA.

1. _____

2. _____

3. _____

7C. What other types of problems are thought to cause CSA?

_____

_____

_____

_____

Think About This:

How does sleeping at a high altitude cause CSA?

NATIONAL BOARD FOR RESPIRATORY CARE (NBRC)–TYPE QUESTIONS

1. The appearance of sleep spindles and K-complexes on a sleeper's electroencephalogram indicates what non-REM sleep stage?
   A. Stage 1
   B. Stage 2
   C. Stage 3
   D. Stage 4

2. The type of electroencephalographic waveform that is indicative of REM sleep is which of the following?
   A. Alpha waves
   B. Beta waves
   C. Delta waves
   D. Theta waves

3. The key to recognizing obstructive sleep apnea when the results of a sleep study are analyzed is which of the following?
   A. No airflow and no respiratory effort
   B. No airflow with increasing respiratory effort
   C. Reduced airflow with minimal respiratory effort
   D. No airflow with no or minimal respiratory effort

4. The physiologic consequences of obstructive sleep apnea include all of the following except
   A. Tachycardia
   B. Acute hypercapnia
   C. Cardiac arrhythmias
   D. Systemic hypertension

5. To establish the diagnosis of sleep apnea, the minimum number of apneic events that have to occur per hour is
   A. 3
   B. 5
   C. 7
   D. 9

6. During which stage of sleep is the threshold for arousability to respiratory stimuli low?
   A. Non-REM stage 2
   B. Non-REM stage 3
   C. Non-REM stage 4
   D. REM sleep

7. High-voltage, slow-wave electroencephalographic activity, absence of eye movements, and tonic electromyographic activity are present during which of the following sleep stages?
   A. Stage W
   B. Non-REM stage 2
   C. Non-REM stage 3
   D. REM sleep

8. During which stage of sleep does breathing normally become irregular?
   A. Stage W
   B. Non-REM stage 2
   C. Non-REM stage 3
   D. REM sleep

9. The variables that are measured during a sleep screening are which of the following?
   (1) Pulse oximetry oxygen saturation (SpO_2)
   (2) Tibialis electromyographic results
   (3) Diaphragm electromyographic results
   (4) The results of Holter monitoring electrocardiography
   A. 1 and 4 only
   B. 1, 2, and 4 only
   C. 2, 3, and 4 only
   D. 2 and 4 only

10. Which of the following could be a cause of central sleep apnea?
    A. Nuchal obesity
    B. Tonsillar enlargement
    C. Myasthenia gravis
    D. Systemic hypertension

12 Introduction to Ventilators

Upon completion of this chapter, you will be able to:
1. List the two primary power sources used in mechanical ventilators.
2. Compare and contrast *negative-pressure ventilation* and *positive-pressure ventilation*.
3. Explain how a *closed-loop ventilator system* can perform self-adjustment.
4. Define *volume* and *pressure ventilation*.
5. Provide three additional names for *pressure ventilation* and *volume ventilation*.
6. Name the *flow-control valve* found on most intensive care unit (ICU) ventilators.
7. Explain the two fundamental principles of *fluidics*.
8. Evaluate available *positive end-expiratory pressure* (PEEP) valves to determine whether a *flow resistor* or a *threshold resistor* is being used.
9. Troubleshoot a *Downs continuous positive airway pressure (CPAP) system*.
10. Describe the four phases of a breath.
11. Explain how pressure-, flow-, and volume-triggering mechanisms work to begin the inspiratory phase of a breath.
12. Identify the scalars for *time-triggered, volume-* or *pressure-limited, time-cycled breaths*.
13. Identify a pressure-time scalar showing patient triggering.
14. Apply Chatburn's classification for ventilator modes.
15. Explain the concept of having an adjustable flow drop-off feature for ending inspiration in *pressure-support ventilation*.
16. Define the modes of ventilation by their *triggering, limiting* (controlling), and *cycling* mechanisms.
17. Describe the six targeting schemes.
18. List examples of modes in each of the six targeting schemes.
19. List the five common methods of delivering *high-frequency ventilation*.

"Breathe. Let go. And remind yourself that this very moment is the only one you know you have for sure."
Oprah Winfrey

ACHIEVING THE OBJECTIVES

1. List the two primary power sources used in mechanical ventilators. (IIA6a)

1A. What is the range of gas power necessary to run a pneumatically powered ventilator?

_____

_____

1B. How does a pneumatic ventilator lower the source pressure to operating pressure?

_____

_____

1C. Name the two types of pneumatically powered ventilators.

(1) _____

(2) _____

1D. What types of ventilators use alternating current to power their internal components?

_____

_____

1E. What is the most common type of intensive care unit (ICU) ventilator used today?

_____

_____

1F. The power sources for these ICU ventilators include

_____

_____.

Think About This:

Which type of ventilator should be used during magnetic resonance imaging (MRI)?

2. Compare and contrast negative-pressure and positive-pressure ventilation. (IIA6a)

2A. For gas to flow, what must exist?

_____

_____

2B. During normal spontaneous breathing, what initiates inspiration?

_____

_____

2C. What is the major muscle of ventilation?

_____

_____

2D. What causes gas to move into the lungs during normal spontaneous breathing?

_____

_____

_____

2E. What causes expiration during normal spontaneous breathing?

_____

_____

_____

2F. How do negative-pressure ventilators cause gas to enter the lungs?

_____

_____

_____

_____

_____

_____

2G. What causes air to flow out of the patient's lungs during negative-pressure ventilation?

_____

_____

_____

_____

_____

2H. Name two types of negative-pressure ventilators.

(1) _____

(2) _____

2I. What causes inspiration during positive-pressure ventilation?

_____

_____

_____

_____

_____

2J. Which form of ventilation is most physiologic?

_____

_____

2K. Which type of ventilation is most commonly used today?

_____

_____

2L. What is the most common example of a combined-pressure device?

_____

Think About This:

How can a vacuum cleaner become a ventilator?

3. Explain how a closed-loop ventilator system can perform self-adjustment. (IIA6a)

3A. What are the characteristics of an *open-loop ventilator system*?

_____

_____.

3B. List two other terms for a *closed-loop ventilator system*.

(1) _____

(2) _____

3C. What specific type of hardware is used to control the function of a closed-loop ventilator system?

_____

_____

3D. What allows a closed-loop ventilator system to perform self-adjustments?

_____

_____

3E. A patient who is breathing spontaneously through a mechanical ventilator becomes apneic. The ventilator alarm rings. What type of ventilator system is this?

_____

_____

3F. A patient who is breathing spontaneously through a mechanical ventilator becomes apneic. The ventilator alarm rings and begins to ventilate the patient. What type of ventilator system is this?

_____

_____

Think About This:
What closed-loop ventilator systems do you use in everyday life?

4. Define volume and pressure ventilation. (IIA6a)

4A. What is a control variable?

_____

_____

4B. Name the three main control variables.

1. _____

2. _____

3. _____

4C. In the clinical setting, what are the two variables that are most commonly controlled?

(1) _____

(2) _____

4D. When volume is the control variable, what happens to the pressure if there is a change in the patient's lung characteristics?

_____

_____

4E. When pressure is the control variable, what happens to the volume and flow if there is a change in the patient's lung characteristics?

_____

_____

4F. What type of ventilation controls the volume variable?

_____

_____

4G. What type of ventilation controls the pressure variable?

_____

_____

139

Think About This:

Which type of ventilation will protect the lungs best?

5. Provide three additional names for pressure and volume ventilation. (IIA6a)

5A. What are the three alternative terms for *volume-targeted ventilation*?

1. _____

2. _____

3. _____

5B. What are the three alternative terms for *pressure-targeted ventilation*?

1. _____

2. _____

3. _____

Think About This:

Can you think of any other industry in which many names have the same meaning and thereby cause so much confusion?

6. Name the flow control valve found on most ICU ventilators. (IIA6a)

6A. What type of device responds rapidly and has precise control over the exact pattern of gas and pressure?

_____

_____

6B. List the three types of flow-controlling valves.

1. _____

2. _____

3. _____

6C. What type of flow-control valve is used in current ICU ventilators?

_____

_____

6D. How do proportional solenoid valves control flow?

_____

_____

_____

6E. Which type of device is based on the principle of physics that concerns electricity and magnetism?

_____

_____

_____

6F. What device measures the flow and volume that pass across a proportional solenoid valve?

_____

_____

6G. Name three ICU ventilators in which a proportional solenoid valve is used.

1. _____

2. _____

3. _____

Think About This:

Will MRI interfere with the operation of ventilator drive mechanisms?

7. Explain the two fundamental principles of fluidics. (IIA6a)

7A. The characteristic of fluidic-operated ventilators that makes them suitable to be used for a patient during MRI is that they

_____

_____

7B. Another name for the *Coanda effect* is

_____

_____

7C. Describe what is shown in Figure 12-1.

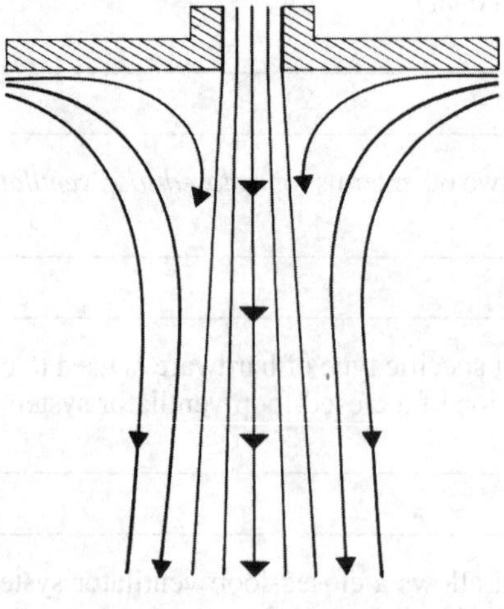

FIGURE 12-1
(From Dupuis YC: *Ventilators: theory and clinical application,* ed 2, St Louis, 1992, Mosby.)

_____

_____

_____

7D. What happens to the jet stream when there is a wall on one side of it?

_____

_____

_____

_____

7E. Describe the phenomenon of beam deflection.

_____

_____

_____

Think About This:

What other applications does the Coanda effect have?

8. Evaluate available positive end-expiratory pressure (PEEP) valves to determine whether a flow resistor or a threshold resistor is being used. (IIA11c)

8A. Expiratory retard can be created by what type of expiratory valve?

_____

_____

8B. Which type of expiratory valve can accommodate high expiratory flow without creating high pressure?

_____

_____

8C. What type of expiratory valve is used in a positive expiratory pressure (PEP) mask?

_____

_____

8D. Why are flow resistors not commonly used for expiratory valves in ventilators?

_____

_____

_____

8E. Why are threshold resistors more commonly used as ventilator expiratory valves?

_____

_____

_____

8F. Identify the type of expiratory valve in Figure 12-2.

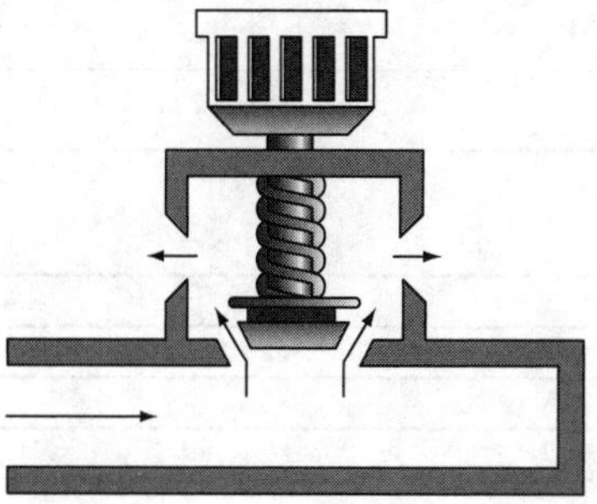

FIGURE 12-2
(Modified from Pilbeam SP, ed: *Mechanical ventilation: physiological and clinical applications,* ed 2, St Louis, 1992, Mosby.)

_____

_____

8G. What type of ventilator has the expiratory valve depicted in Figure 12-2?

_____

_____

8H. Identify the type of expiratory valve depicted in Figure 12-3.

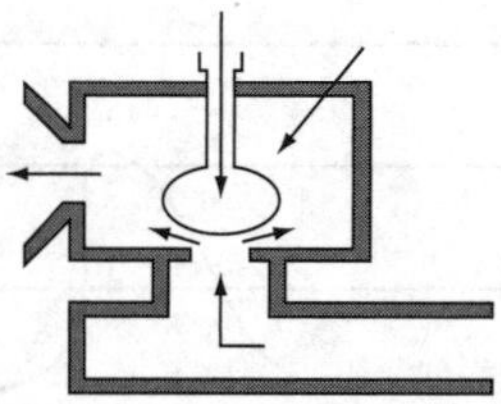

FIGURE 12-3
(Modified from Pilbeam SP, ed: *Mechanical ventilation: physiological and clinical applications,* ed 2, St Louis, 1992, Mosby.)

_____

_____

8I. What type of valve is an electromagnetic valve?

_____

_____

8J. Identify the type of expiratory valve that produces the pressure-time curve in Figure 12-4.

_____

_____

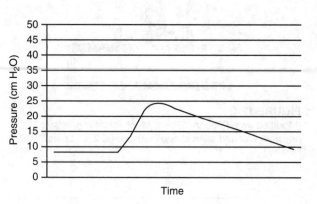

FIGURE 12-4

8K. Identify the type of expiratory valve that produces the pressure-time curve in Figure 12-5.

_____

_____

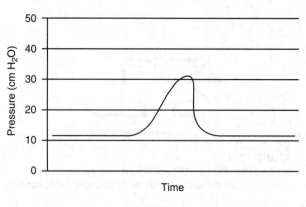

FIGURE 12-5

Think About This:

What effects does expiratory resistance have on the inspiratory work of breathing?

9. Troubleshoot a Downs CPAP system. (IIA2)

9A. What is the purpose of the safety pressure-release valve on a CPAP system?

_____

_____

9B. How is the safety pressure-release valve set?

_____

_____

9C. During the use of a freestanding CPAP unit, the safety pop-in valve is being opened on every breath. What is the most likely problem in this situation?

_____

_____

9D. A patient is using a freestanding CPAP system with a low-pressure alarm that is actively alarming. What is the most likely problem?

_____

_____

Think About This:

Why is CPAP used for sleep apnea?

10. Describe the four phases of a breath.

10A. What is the definition of the term *breath*?

_____

_____

10B. What is the formula for total cycle time?

_____

_____

10C. The first breath phase is

_____

_____

10D. The second breath phase is

_____

_____

10E. The third breath phase is

_____

_____

10F. The fourth breath phase is

_____

_____

10G. Define *phase variable*.

_____

_____

10H. What phase variable begins inspiration?

_____

10I. Define *cycle variable*.

_____

_____

10J. What are the two most common control variables?

(1) _____

(2) _____

10K. Define the term *limit variable*.

_____

_____

10L. During expiration, what two variables can be controlled?

(1) _____

(2) _____

Think About This:

What controls the four variables of a spontaneous breath?

11. Explain how pressure-, flow-, and volume-triggering mechanisms work to begin the inspiratory phase of a breath. (IIA6a)

11A. How does a patient pressure-trigger inspiration?

_____

_____

11B. What is baseline pressure?

_____

_____

11C. In what three places is pressure measured in the ventilator circuit?

(1) _____

(2) _____

(3) _____

11D. What device measures pressure?

_____

_____

11E. The pressure baseline is set at 5 cm H_2O, and the sensitivity is set at 1.5 cm H_2O. At what pressure will the ventilator be pressure-triggered?

_____

_____

11F. Define *base flow* or *bias flow*.

_____

_____

11G. What three factors determine the flow-trigger setting?

(1) _____

(2) _____

(3) _____

11H. Describe how the flow trigger works.

_____

_____

_____

_____

11I. The base flow is set at 5 L/min, and the flow trigger is set at 2 L/min. The base flow must drop to what value before the ventilator will flow-trigger?

_____

_____

11J. Explain how the volume trigger operates.

_____

_____

Think About This:

How does the patient's trigger effort affect work of breathing?

12. Identify the scalars for time-triggered, volume- or pressure-limited, and time-cycled breaths. (IIID3)

Questions 12A through 12G refer to Figure 12-6.

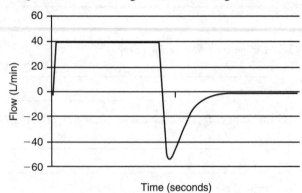

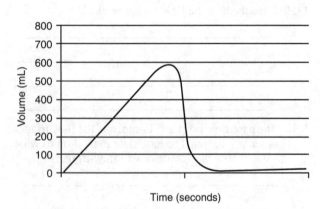

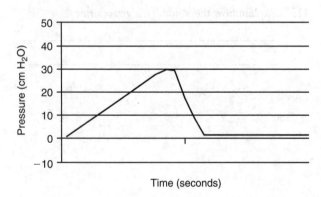

FIGURE 12-6

12A. The trigger in Figure 12-6 is

_____.

12B. What variable is limited in Figure 12-6?

_____

12C. What is the cycle variable in Figure 12-6?

_____

12D. What type of flow waveform is shown in Figure 12-6?

_____

12E. The peak inspiratory pressure in Figure 12-6 is

_____.

12F. What is the peak flow setting in Figure 12-6?

_____

12G. What volume is delivered in Figure 12-6?

_____

Questions 12H through 12N refer to Figure 12-7.

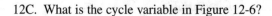

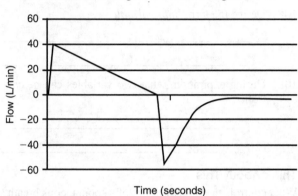

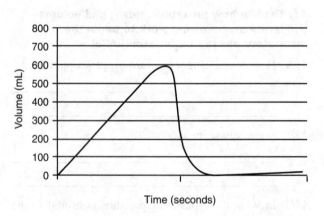

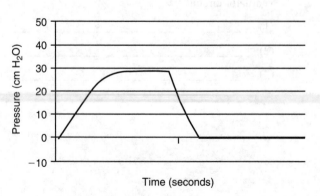

FIGURE 12-7

12H. The trigger in Figure 12-7 is

_____.

12I. What variable is limited in Figure 12-7?

_____

12J. What is the cycle variable in Figure 12-7?

_____

12K. What type of flow waveform is shown in Figure 12-7?

_____

12L. The peak inspiratory pressure in Figure 12-7 is

_____.

12M. What is the peak flow setting in Figure 12-7?

_____

12N. What volume is delivered in Figure 12-7?

_____

Think About This:

Which do you think is the most important scalar to monitor and why?

13. Identify a pressure-time scalar showing patient triggering. (IIID3)

13A. Use Figure 12-8 to draw and label a pressure–time curve for a volume-cycled breath with a baseline of +5 cm H_2O, a trigger of –1 cm H_2O, and a peak inspiratory pressure of 25 cm H_2O.

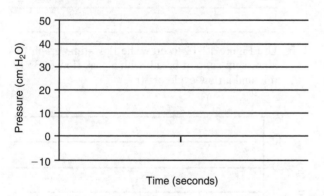

FIGURE 12-8

13B. Use Figure 12-9 to draw and label a pressure time curve for a pressure-limited breath with a baseline of +10 cm H_2O, a trigger of 1.5 cm H_2O, and a pressure limit setting of 30 cm H_2O.

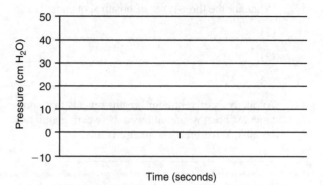

FIGURE 12-9

13C. Circle the pressure-triggered breaths in Figure 12-10.

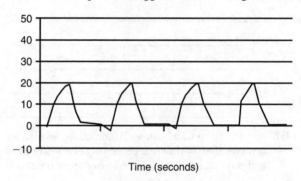

FIGURE 12-10

Think About This:

What effect does intrinsic PEEP have on pressure triggering?

14. Apply Chatburn's classification for ventilator modes. (IIA6a)

14A. A mode description according to Chatburn is

_____

_____.

14B. What is the key point of the equation of motion?

_____

_____

14C. What are the two main breath-control variables?

(1) _____

(2) _____

14D. In pressure control, _____ is constant, and _____ can vary. In volume control, _____ is constant, and _____ can vary.

14E. What are the three types of breath sequences?

(1) _____

(2) _____

(3) _____

14F. An analysis of ventilator breaths reveals that spontaneous breaths are allowed between mandatory breaths. What breath sequence is this?

_____

_____

14G. Describe the three main categories of control types used in mechanical ventilation.

(1) _____

_____

(2) _____

_____

(3) _____

_____

14H. According to Chatburn's classification, level 1 for a mode that is time-triggered or patient-triggered and provides volume-targeted mandatory breaths is

_____

_____.

14I. According to Chatburn's classification, level 1 for a mode that allows the patient to breathe spontaneously between mandatory ventilator breaths that are pressure-targeted is

_____

_____.

14J. According to Chatburn's classification, level 1 for a mode that provides pressure-targeted spontaneous breaths is

_____

_____

Think About This:

Can you think of items in your everyday life that do the same thing but have different names?

15. Explain the concept of having an adjustable flow drop-off feature for ending inspiration in pressure-support ventilation. (IIA6a)

15A. According to Chatburn's classification, level 1 for pressure-support ventilation is

_____

_____.

15B. What are the phase variables for pressure-support ventilation?

_____

_____

15C. Describe the flow–time curve for pressure-support ventilation.

_____

_____

15D. What is the reason for the specific appearance of the flow–time curve?

_____

_____

15E. Which ventilators allow the operator to change the cycle level (percentage of flow)?

_____

_____

15F. Use Figure 12-11 to draw the flow–time graph for a pressure-support breath with a peak flow of 35 L/min and a flow cycle of 30%.

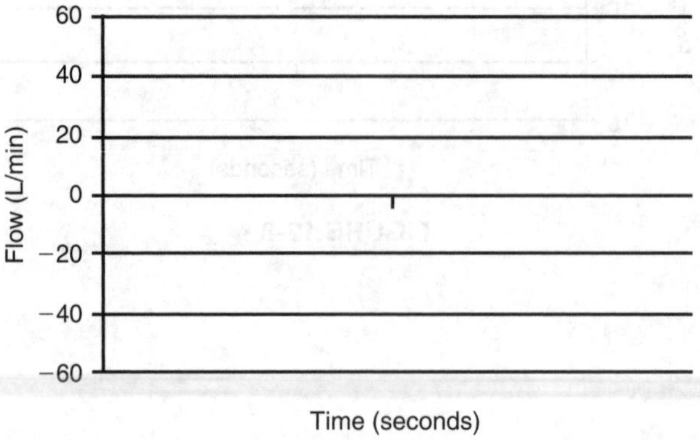

FIGURE 12-11

15G. What happens to the flow cycle if there is a leak in the system during the delivery of a pressure-support breath?

_____

_____

_____

_____

_____

15H. During pressure-support ventilation, the patient coughs. What happens with the ventilator in this situation?

_____

_____

_____

15I. What three factors determine how much volume will be delivered during a pressure-support breath?

(1) _____

(2) _____

(3) _____

15J. Why would a patient with a nasal intubation benefit from the use of pressure-support ventilation while breathing spontaneously?

_____

_____

_____

Think About This:

Which types of patients should have their flow cycles set higher?

16. Define the modes of ventilation by their triggering, limiting (controlling), and cycling mechanisms. (IIA6a)

Questions 16A through 16D refer to Figure 12-12.

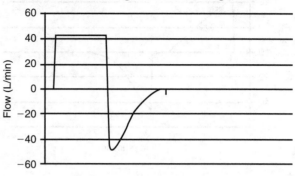

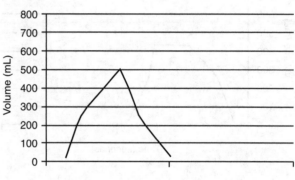

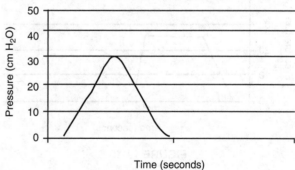

FIGURE 12-12

16A. What variable is the trigger in Figure 12-12?

_____

16B. What variable is the limit in Figure 12-12?

_____

16C. What variable is the cycle in Figure 12-12?

_____

16D. What mode of ventilation is shown in Figure 12-12?

_____

Questions 16E through 16H refer to Figure 12-13.

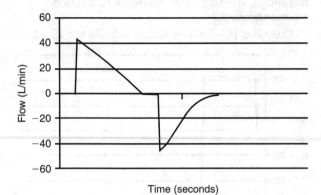

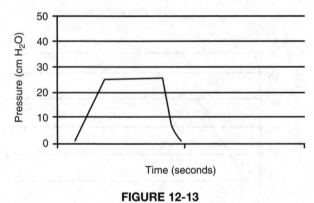

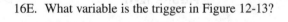

FIGURE 12-13

Questions 16I through 16M refer to Figure 12-14.

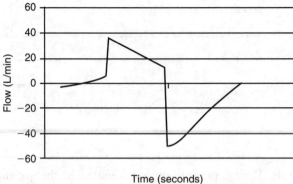

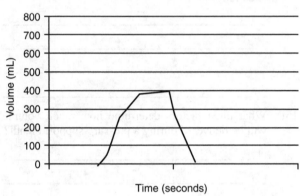

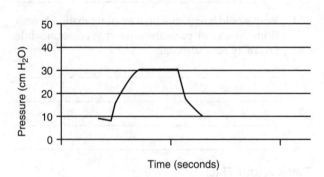

FIGURE 12-14

16E. What variable is the trigger in Figure 12-13?

_____

16F. What variable is the limit in Figure 12-13?

_____

16G. What variable is the cycle in Figure 12-13?

_____

16H. What mode of ventilation is shown in Figure 12-13?

_____

16I. What variable is the trigger in Figure 12-14?

_____

16J. What variable is the limit in Figure 12-14?

_____

16K. What variable is the cycle in Figure 12-14?

_____

16L. What is the baseline pressure?

_____

16M. What mode of ventilation is shown in Figure 12-14?

_____

16N. "Flow-triggered, pressure-limited, flow-cycled breaths with intermittent flow" or "time-triggered, pressure-limited, time-cycled breaths" describes what mode of ventilation?

_____

_____

Think About This:

Trigger, limit, cycle = start, contain, end.

17. Describe the six targeting schemes. (IIA6a)

17A. List the six targeting schemes.

(1) _____ (4) _____

(2) _____ (5) _____

(3) _____ (6) _____

17B. The target scheme in which the ventilator matches a constant operator pre-set input value is termed

_____

17C. Describe the characteristics of a duel-targeted breath.

_____

_____

_____

17D. The target scheme in which the ventilator output (e.g., tidal volume or pressure) automatically follows a varying output (e.g., lung mechanics) is termed

_____

17E. Provide an example of an adaptive target scheme.

_____

_____

_____

17F. In which target scheme does the Otis formula serve as the model of system behavior?

_____

17G. The term for the target scheme in which set points are automatically adjusted to maintain a patient's "respiratory zone of comfort" is

_____

Think About This:

Will ventilators with the intelligent target scheme replace respiratory therapists?

18. List examples of modes in each of the six targeting schemes. (IIA6a)

18A. Complete the table below.

Target Scheme	Mode	Ventilator

Think About This:

Is it necessary to memorize the modes found on each ventilator?

19. List the five common methods of delivering high-frequency ventilation. (IIA6c)

19A. Define *high-frequency ventilation*.

_____

_____

19B. Define *high-frequency positive-pressure ventilation*.

_____

_____

_____

19C. What rates are used in high-frequency jet ventilation?

_____

19D. What is the operational principle of high-frequency jet ventilation?

_____

_____

_____

19E. Identify the components of a triple-lumen endotracheal tube.

_____

_____

_____

_____

19F. What rates are used in high-frequency oscillatory ventilation (HFOV)?

_____

19G. How is gas moved during HFOV?

_____

_____

_____

_____

19H. What characteristics does a high-frequency percussive ventilation (HFPV) device have?

_____

_____

_____

_____

19I. What is the operating principle of HFPV?

_____

_____

_____

19J. Identify the clinical applications for HFPV.

_____

_____

_____

Think About This:

Is high-frequency ventilation more advantageous than conventional ventilation for adults in respiratory failure?

NATIONAL BOARD FOR RESPIRATORY CARE (NBRC)–TYPE QUESTIONS

1. Active expiration occurs in which ventilator mode?
   A. Proportional assist ventilation
   B. High-frequency jet ventilation
   C. Airway pressure-release ventilation
   D. High-frequency oscillatory ventilation

2. A patient receiving mask CPAP, 7.5 cm H_2O, via a freestanding system appears to be in distress. The patient is using accessory muscles and is diaphoretic. The manometer is fluctuating between –5 cm H_2O on inspiration and 7.5 cm H_2O on expiration. The most apparent cause of the patient's distress is which of the following?
   A. Leak in the system
   B. Improper mask fitting
   C. Inadequate flow rate
   D. Obstruction of the threshold resistor

3. The amount of time for a pressure-targeted ventilator breath to reach the set pressure is known as which of the following?
   A. Rise time
   B. Inspiratory time
   C. Total cycle time
   D. Inspiratory hold

4. Which of the following is the mode in which the ventilator adjusts either the mandatory rate or level of pressure support to achieve target minute ventilation?
   A. Proportional assist ventilation
   B. Mandatory minute ventilation
   C. Airway pressure-release ventilation
   D. Pressure augmentation

5. What type of flow–time curve will be created by means of a linear-drive piston?
   A. Ascending ramp
   B. Descending ramp
   C. Rectangular
   D. Sine wave

6. The baseline pressure is elevated but is periodically released to a lower level for a very brief period. This statement describes which ventilator mode?
   A. Bilevel positive airway pressure (BiPAP)
   B. Pressure-controlled inverse-ratio ventilation (PCIRV)
   C. Airway pressure-release ventilation (APRV)
   D. Mandatory minute ventilation (MMV)

7. Patient discomfort from rapid gas flow during pressure-targeted ventilation may be alleviated by which of the following adjustments to the ventilator?
   A. Increasing inspiratory time
   B. Increasing rise time
   C. Decreasing expiratory time
   D. Decreasing total cycle time

8. The flow cycle setting for a pressure-supported breath, with a peak flow of 30 L/min, that will allow enough time for a visible plateau on the pressure-time curve is which of the following?
   A. 10 L/min
   B. 17% of peak flow
   C. 20 L/min
   D. 57% of peak flow

9. A flow–time curve that does not return to 0 before the next mandatory breath indicates which of the following?
   A. Flow-triggering
   B. Auto-PEEP
   C. Flow-cycling
   D. A system leak

10. A ventilator mode used prophylactically in patients with thermal airway injury to help prevent pneumonia and atelectasis is which of the following?
    A. APRV
    B. HFPV
    C. High-frequency jet ventilation
    D. PCIRV

13 Mechanical Ventilators: General-Use Devices

This chapter has been designed in a slightly different manner than other chapters in the workbook. The chapter is divided into the various ventilator sections, each with its own set of learning objectives, as identified in the textbook, short-answer questions, fill-in questions, and *National Board for Respiratory Care* (NBRC)–type multiple-choice questions. The *"Think About This"* also appears at the end of each ventilator section.

"The cardinal virtue of a teacher (is) to protect the pupil from his own influence."
Ralph Waldo Emerson

I. Carefusion AVEA

Upon completion of this section, you will be able to:
1. Identify the icons and waveforms on the main screen.
2. Describe visual and audible alarm signals.
3. Describe the purpose of each of the extended settings.
4. List the differences between adult and neonatal modes of ventilation?

ACHIEVING THE OBJECTIVES

1. Identify the icons and waveforms on the main screen. (IIA6a)
Refer to Figure 13-1 to answer Questions 1A through 1D.

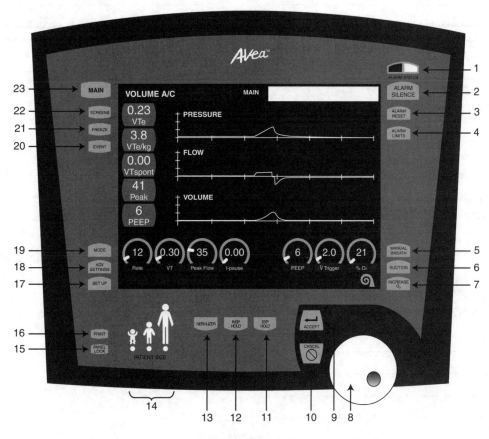

FIGURE 13-1

1A. Where is the current mode displayed on the main screen?

_____

_____

1B. Identify the primary breath controls that are displayed in the volume A/C mode of ventilation.

_____

_____

_____

1C. Which monitored parameters are displayed on the main screen?

_____

_____

_____

_____

_____

_____

1D. Which waveforms are being displayed on the main screen?

_____

_____

_____

2. Describe visual and audible alarm signals. (IIA6a)

2A. What is the location of the ALARM STATUS membrane button?

_____

_____

2B. How are alarm messages ordered in the ALARM STATUS drop-down display?

_____

_____

2C. Which alarms cause the safety valve to open?

_____

_____

_____

3. Describe the purpose of each of the extended settings. (IIA6a)

3A. What do the extended settings allow the clinician to do?

_____

_____

3B. Describe machine volume (MACH VOL) and its purpose.

_____

_____

_____

_____

_____

_____

_____

_____

3C. What does "PSV" Tmax limit?

_____

_____

_____

_____

3D. How does the independent lung ventilation (ILV) feature function?

_____

_____

_____

4. List the differences beween adult and neonatal modes of ventilation. (IIA6a)

4A. What modes in addition to standard neonatal modes are available on the CareFusion AVEA?

_____

_____

4B. What monitoring device is recommended when the CareFusion AVEA is used for neonatal ventilation?

_____

_____

_____

_____

_____

_____

Think About This:

What are the steps in the development of a new ventilator mode?

NATIONAL BOARD FOR RESPIRATORY CARE (NBRC)–TYPE QUESTIONS
CAREFUSION AVEA

1. *A*pnea *b*ack-up *v*entilation (ABV) is active on the CareFusion AVEA ventilator during the use of which of the following modes of ventilation?
   1. Volume assist/control (A/C)
   2. Pressure synchronized intermittent mandatory ventilation (SIMV)
   3. Airway pressure-release ventilation (APRV)/ BiPhasic
   4. Pressure-regulated volume control (PRVC) A/C
      A. 1 and 2 only
      B. 2 and 3 only
      C. 3 and 4 only
      D. 1 and 4 only

2. Calculate the flow at which the ventilator will cycle when the CareFusion AVEA ventilator is in the pressure A/C mode, the flow cycle is set at 40%, and the peak inspiratory flow is 45 L/min.
   A. 18 L/min
   B. 20 L/min
   C. 25 L/min
   D. Flow-cycling is available only during spontaneous breaths.

3. Use of Vsync on the CareFusion AVEA ventilator will change volume breaths into which of the following?
   A. Pressure-limited, volume-targeted breaths
   B. Volume-limited, pressure-targeted breaths
   C. Pressure-limited, flow-cycled breaths
   D. Volume-limited, time-cycled breaths

4. An adult is being ventilated with the CareFusion AVEA in the PRVC mode. The ventilator is not delivering the set volume. The ventilator will do which of the following?
   A. Initiate ABV.
   B. Change over to volume-targeted ventilation.
   C. Produce an audible and visual high-priority alarm.
   D. Increase pressure by 3 cm H_2O to achieve the minimum volume.

5. The CareFusion AVEA offers all of the following patient monitoring features EXCEPT:
   A. Esophageal pressure
   B. Diaphragmatic activity
   C. Tracheal pressure
   D. Proximal airway pressure

II. Dräger EvitaXL

LEARNING OBJECTIVES

Upon completion of this section, you will be able to:
1. Identify the specific areas of the Dräger EvitaXL front control panel.
2. List the modes of ventilation available for the Dräger EvitaXL.
3. List the differences between adult and neonatal modes of ventilation?

ACHIEVING THE OBJECTIVES

1. Identify the specific areas of the Dräger EvitaXL front control panel. (IIA6a)

Refer to Figure 13-2 to answer Questions 1A through 1C.

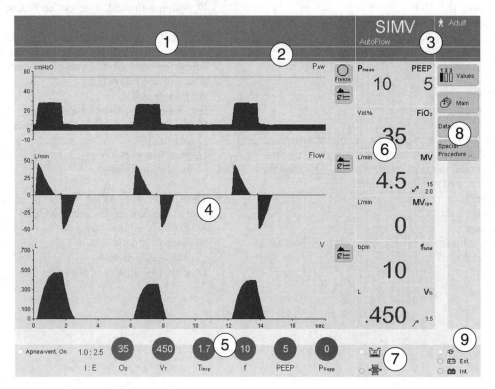

FIGURE 13-2
(Courtesy Dräger Medical, Telford, PA)

1A. Name the peripheral control keys, from top to bottom, located on the right side of the screen.

_____

_____

_____

_____

1B. Where is the control knob located?

_____

_____

1C. Where are the set ventilation parameters for the active ventilation mode located?

_____

_____

2. List the modes of ventilation available for the Dräger EvitaXL. (IIA6a)

_____

_____

_____

_____

_____

3. List the differences between adult and neonatal modes of ventilation? (IIA6a)

3A. What is required to use the Dräger EvitaXL for neonatal ventilation?

_____

_____

_____

3B. What modes of ventilation are available for neonatal patients?

_____

_____

_____

_____

_____

Think About This:

How long does it take for a new ventilator to go from the research and design stage to operation in the clinical setting?

Name _____

Date _____

NATIONAL BOARD FOR RESPIRATORY CARE (NBRC)–TYPE QUESTIONS
DRÄGER EVITAXL

1. Which of the following functions automatically increases the level of PEEP for two consecutive breaths while the ventilator is in the CMV mode?
   A. Sigh
   B. Automatic tube compensation (ATC)
   C. Occlusion pressure
   D. Low-flow PV-loop

2. Which of the following is used to measure auto-PEEP on the Dräger EvitaXL?
   A. Inspiratory hold
   B. Expiratory hold
   C. Occlusion pressure
   D. Manual inspiration

3. During SmartCare a patient's spontaneous respiratory rate increases from 20 to 35 breaths/min. The Dräger EvitaXL will respond by doing which of the following?
   A. Switching to SIMV
   B. Increasing tidal volume
   C. Sounding an alarm for high respiratory rate
   D. Increasing pressure support by 4 mbar

4. Which of the following is a pressure-limited, volume-targeted dual-control mode of ventilation in which the Dräger EvitaXL can adjust pressure to achieve the set volume?
   A. PLV
   B. PCV+
   C. APRV
   D. AutoFlow

5. During MMV using the Dräger EvitaXL, what will occur if the patient's spontaneous breathing drops below the pre-selected MMV setting?
   A. The apnea alarm sounds.
   B. A mandatory breath is delivered.
   C. The pressure support is increased.
   D. The PEEP is increased.

III. Dräger Evita Infinity V500 and N500

LEARNING OBJECTIVES

Upon completion of this section, you will be able to:
1. Identify the specific areas of the Dräger Evita Infinity V500 front control panel.
2. List the modes of ventilation available for the Dräger Evita Infinity V500.
3. List two extended monitoring features on the V500.
4. Compare adult and neonatal ventilation on the V500 and N500.

1. Identify the specific areas of the Dräger Evita Infinity V500 front control panel. (IIA6a)

Refer to Figure 13-3 to answer questions 1A through 1C.

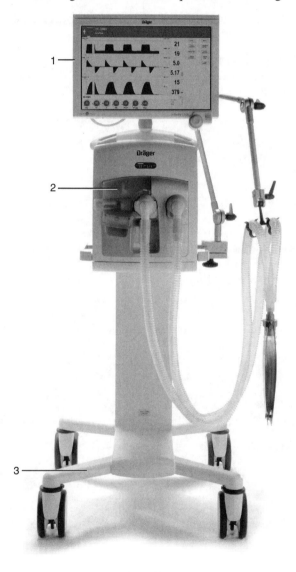

FIGURE 13-3

1A. Where are the monitored parameters displayed on the screen?

_____

_____

1B. Where is the control knob located?

_____

_____

1C. Where are the set ventilator parameters for the active ventilation mode located?

_____

_____

2. List the modes available for the Dräger Evita Infinity V500. (IIA6a)

_____

_____

_____

3. List the two extended monitoring features on the V500. (IIA6a)

3A. What does *Smart Pulmonary View* provide for the clinician?_____

_____

3B. What is the purpose of the Low Flow PV Loop?_____

_____

4. Compare adult and neonatal modes of ventilation on the V500 and N500. (IIA6a)

4A. What is required to use the V500 for neonatal ventilation?_____

_____

4B. What modes of ventilation are available for neonatal patients?_____

_____

Think About This:

What makes a ventilator obsolete?

NATIONAL BOARD FOR RESPIRATORY CARE (NBRC)–TYPE QUESTIONS
DRÄGER EVITA INFINITY V500

1. What does the Dräger Evita Infinity V500 ventilator compare when utilizing the automatic leakage compensation feature?
   A. Delivered volume and exhaled volume
   B. Delivered flow and exhaled flow
   C. Delivered pressure and exhaled pressure
   D. Inspiratory time and expiratory time

2. Which of the following is a closed-loop form of ventilation designed to shorten weaning time?
   A. APRV
   B. BiPAP
   C. SmartCare
   D. AutoFlow

3. What feature available on the Dräger Evita Infinity V500 is used to compensate for airway resistance associated with small artificial airways?
   A. ATC
   B. PPS
   C. ALC
   D. PCV

4. What mode available on the Dräger Evita Infinity V500 adjusts pressure support in proportion to the patient's breathing effort?
   A. APRV
   B. PSV
   C. SIMV/PS
   D. PPS

5. The pressure measured during an expiratory hold maneuver is
   A. P_{peak}
   B. Auto-PEEP
   C. P_{plat}
   D. P_{max}

IV. GE Healthcare Engström Carestation

Upon completion of this section, you will be able to:
1. List the standard modes of ventilation found on the GE Healthcare Engström Carestation (GE Carestation).
2. Describe the function of the airway resistance compensation (ARC) extended feature.
3. List measurements obtained with the gas modules.
4. Describe measurements obtained with the FRC INview module.
5. Describe options available for neonatal ventilation.

1. List the standard modes of ventilation found on the GE Carestation. (IIA6a)

_____

_____

_____

_____

_____

2. Describe the function of the ARC extended feature. (IIA6a)

_____

_____

_____

_____

3. List measurements obtained with the gas modules. (IIA6a)

_____

_____

_____

4. Describe measurements obtained with the FRC INview module. (IIA6a)

_____

_____

_____

5. Describe options available for neonatal ventilation. (IIA6a)

5A. What is used to monitor volumes during neonatal ventilation?

_____

_____

_____

5B. What modes are available for neonatal ventilation?

_____

_____

_____

_____

Think About This:
Why are computerized ventilators easier to upgrade?

NATIONAL BOARD FOR RESPIRATORY CARE (NBRC)–TYPE QUESTIONS
GE HEALTHCARE ENGSTRÖM CARESTATION

1. The INview ventilator calculations available on the GE Carestation include which of the following?
   1. P_AO_2
   2. V_d/V_t
   3. A-a DO_2
   4. CvO_2
   - A. 1 only
   - B. 1 and 2 only
   - C. 1, 2, and 3 only
   - D. 3 and 4 only

2. Which of the following is needed to utilize the SpiroDynamics monitoring feature on the GE Carestation?
   - A. Esophageal catheter
   - B. Tracheal catheter
   - C. Nasogastric tube
   - D. Diaphragmatic electrode

3. The FRC INview monitoring feature uses which of the following techniques to measure FRC?
   - A. Helium dilution
   - B. Plethysmography
   - C. Direct measurement
   - D. Nitrogen wash-out

4. Which of the following measurements are used to calculate RQ and EE using the metabolic gas monitoring feature on the GE Carestation?
   1. VO_2
   2. P_AO_2
   3. CO
   4. Vco_2
   - A. 1 only
   - B. 1 and 3 only
   - C. 4 only
   - D. 1 and 4 only

5. All of the following spirometry loops are available on the GE Carestation EXCEPT:
   - A. Volume-Time
   - B. Pressure-Volume
   - C. Flow-Volume
   - D. Pressure-Flow

V. Hamilton G5

Upon completion of this section, you will be able to:
1. Identify how control functions are accessed.
2. List the standard measured display of monitoring data.
3. Describe the use of the P/V tool.
4. List the standard modes of ventilation.
5. Describe the function of adaptive support ventilation (ASV).
6. Compare the differences between adult and neonatal modes of ventilation?

ACHIEVING THE OBJECTIVES

1. Identify how control functions are accessed. (IIA6a)

_____

_____

_____

_____

2. List the standard measured display of monitoring data. (IIA6a)

Refer to Figure 13-4 to answer Questions 2A and 2B.

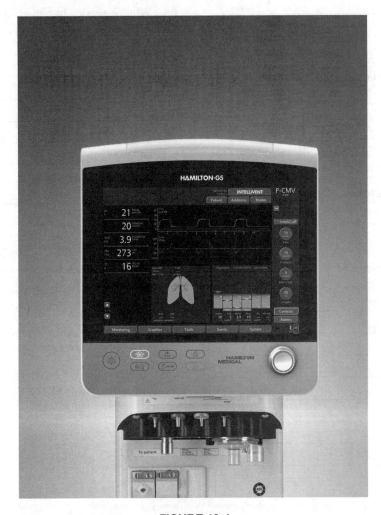

FIGURE 13-4

2A. Identify the main monitoring parameters (MMP) shown in Figure 13-4.

_____

_____

_____

_____

_____

2B. How are the secondary monitoring parameters (SMP) reviewed?

_____

_____

_____

_____

3. Describe the use of the P/V tool. (IIA6a)

3A. What is the function of the P/V tool?

_____

_____

_____

_____

3B. What results are obtained from the P/V tool?

_____

_____

_____

_____

4. List the standard modes of ventilation. (IIA6a)

_____

_____

_____

_____

_____

_____

_____

_____

_____

_____

_____

5. Describe the function of adaptive support ventilation (ASV). (IIA6a)

5A. Describe ASV.

_____

_____

_____

_____

5B. What is the goal of ASV?

_____

_____

_____

_____

_____

_____

6. Compare the differences between adult and neonatal modes of ventilation. (IIA6a)

6A. What is needed to provide neonatal ventilation with the Hamilton G5?

_____

_____

_____

_____

6B. What modes of ventilation are available for neonatal patients?

_____

_____

_____

_____

_____

_____

Think About This:
Can ASV reduce medical errors?

NATIONAL BOARD FOR RESPIRATORY CARE (NBRC)–TYPE QUESTIONS
HAMILTON G5

1. In the CMV-PC + APV mode, the Pmax is set at 32 cm H_2O. Which of the following is the maximum pressure that the Hamilton G5 can use to deliver the targeted volume?
   A. 17 cm H_2O
   B. 22 cm H_2O
   C. 27 cm H_2O
   D. 32 cm H_2O

2. A patient is being ventilated in the ASV mode on the G5. The % Min Vol is 100%; PEEP is 6 cm H_2O; and the spontaneous respiratory rate is 10 breaths/min. An arterial blood gas analysis reveals a pH of 7.28 and a partial pressure of arterial carbon dioxide ($Paco_2$) of 58. Which of the following changes to ASV could correct this problem?
   A. Increase the % Min Vol.
   B. Decrease the % Min Vol.
   C. Decrease PEEP setting.
   D. Increase the set frequency.

3. A patient is being ventilated with the Hamilton G5 at the following settings: (S)CMV frequency, 14 breaths/min; tidal volume, 450 mL; PEEP, 8 cm H_2O. The respiratory therapist activates the sigh function. What is the sigh V_T and rate?
   A. Twice every 50 breaths with 900 mL
   B. Once every 100 breaths with 675 mL
   C. Once every 100 breaths with 900 mL
   D. Twice every 100 breaths at the volume generated by doubling PEEP

4. APRV is similar to which of the following modes on the Hamilton G5?
   A. ASV
   B. DuoPAP
   C. APVcmv
   D. S(CMV)

5. What does the PTP monitoring feature indicate?
   A. The work imposed by the ventilator circuit.
   B. The patient's respiratory drive.
   C. The work by the patient to trigger a breath.
   D. The work imposed by an artificial airway

Chapter **13** Mechanical Ventilators: General-Use Devices

VI. Hamilton C3

Upon completion of this section, you will be able to:
1. List the standard modes of ventilation.
2. Describe how adaptive pressure ventilation (APV) differs from CMV-VC.
3. Describe the function of tube resistance compensation (TRC).
4. Describe how the Hamilton C3 measures alveolar ventilation and calculates dead-space ventilation.
5. Compare the difference between adult and neonatal modes of ventilation?

ACHIEVING THE OBJECTIVES

1. List the standard modes of ventilation. (IIA6a)

_____

_____

_____

_____

_____

2. Describe how adaptive support ventilation (APV) differs from CMV-VC. (IIA6a)

_____

_____

_____

_____

3. Describe the function of tube resistance compensation (TRC). (IIA6a)

_____

_____

_____

_____

4. Describe how the Hamilton C3 measures alveolar ventilation. (IIA6a)

4A. How does the Hamilton C3 measure alveolar ventilation?

_____

_____

4B. How does the Hamilton C3 calculate dead-space ventilation?

_____

_____

5. Compare the difference between adult and neonatal modes of ventilation. (IIA6a)

5A. What is needed to provide neonatal ventilation with the Hamilton C3?

_____

_____

5B. What modes of ventilation are available for the neonatal patient?

_____

_____

Think About This:
Why do ventilators have names?

NATIONAL BOARD FOR RESPIRATORY CARE (NBRC)–TYPE QUESTIONS
HAMILTION C3

1. The apnea alarm trigger time for an adult on the Hamilton C3 ventilator is which of the following?
   A. 10 seconds
   B. 15 seconds
   C. 20 seconds
   D. Operator-selected

2. Which of the following statements is true concerning the Hamilton C3 ventilator?
   A. Nebulizer use will increase the delivered F_IO_2.
   B. The ABV parameters are nonadjustable.
   C. The ventilator can operate for 2 hours on an internal battery.
   D. The lung icon touch pad allows access to tube-resistance compensation.

3. The primary breath type delivered by the Hamilton C3 is?
   A. PSV
   B. VCV
   C. PCV
   D. APV

4. Which of the following parameters on the Hamilton C3 is used to set the pressure above PEEP during controlled breaths?
   A. $P_{control}$
   B. P-ASV
   C. Pause
   D. P_{high}

5. Which of the following are needed to initiate DuoPAP on the Hamilton C3?
   1. T_{high}
   2. V_{target}
   3. T_{low}
   4. P_{low}
   A. 1 and 2 only
   B. 1 and 3 only
   C. 2 and 4 only
   D. 1, 3, and 4 only

VII. Covidien Puritan Bennett (PB) 840

Upon completion of this section, you will be able to:
1. Provide a definition of the parameter settings in the lower screen.
2. List the information contained in the upper screen.
3. Define the modes of ventilation available.
4. Define Proportional Assist Ventilation Plus (PAV+).
5. Compare the differences between adult and neonatal modes of ventilation?

ACHIEVING THE OBJECTIVES

1. Provide a definition of the parameter settings in the lower screen. (IIA6a)

Refer to Figure 13-5 to answer Questions 1A through 1C.

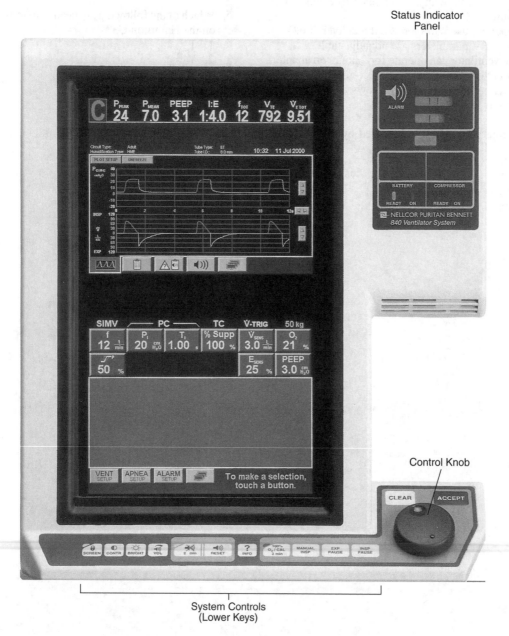

FIGURE 13-5
(Courtesy Covidien Puritan Bennett, Mansfield, CT)

168

1A. List the five areas of the lower screen.

_____

_____

_____

_____

_____

1B. Where do the current set parameters appear on the lower screen?

_____

_____

1C. What parameter settings might appear on the lower screen?

_____

_____

_____

_____

_____

_____

2. List the information contained in the upper screen. (IIA6a)

Refer to Figure 13-6 to answer Questions 2A and 2B.

2A. What areas are contained in the upper screen?

_____

_____

2B. Give examples of monitoring parameters that are displayed at the very top of the screen.

_____

_____

3. Define the modes of ventilation available. (IIA6a)

_____

_____

_____

_____

_____

_____

_____

_____

_____

4. Define Proportional Assist Ventilation Plus (PAV+). (IIA6a)

4A. What is the rationale for PAV+?

_____

_____

_____

4B. How does the ventilator function in PAV+?

_____

_____

4C. What is the level of support (% SUPPORT) available in PAV+?

_____

_____

_____

_____

_____

_____

5. Compare the differences between adult and neonatal modes of ventilation. (IIA6a)

5A. How is neonatal ventilation provided with the Covidien PB 840?

_____

_____

_____

5B. What modes of ventilation are available for the neonatal patient?

_____

_____

Think About This:

Purchasing a ventilator is like purchasing an automobile.

NATIONAL BOARD FOR RESPIRATORY CARE (NBRC)–TYPE QUESTIONS
COVIDIEN PB 840

1. Which of the following describes the function of the expiratory filter?
   1. It humidifies the gas.
   2. It warms the exhaled gas.
   3. It protects the ventilator from microorganisms.
   4. It captures condensation from exhaled gas.
      A. 3 only
      B. 2 and 3 only
      C. 1 and 4 only
      D. 1, 2, 3, and 4

2. Overinflation of the lungs during PAV+ can be caused by which of the following?
   1. Underestimating patient compliance
   2. Overestimating patient compliance
   3. Underestimating airway resistance
   4. Overestimating airway resistance
      A. 1 and 3
      B. 1 and 4
      C. 2 and 3
      D. 2 and 4

3. Calculate the T_E during pressure ventilation when the T_I is locked at 0.85 second and the rate is set at 14 breaths/min.
   A. 1.07 second
   B. 3.44 seconds
   C. 3.98 seconds
   D. 4.19 seconds

4. VS on the Covidien PB 840 is the same as which of the following?
   A. APRV with a volume target
   B. CPAP with a volume target
   C. VC with a pressure target
   D. PSV with a volume target

5. During what modes is rise time percent active for the Covidien PB 840?
   1. PS
   2. VC
   3. PC
   4. SIMV-VC
      A. 1 only
      B. 2 and 3 only
      C. 1 and 3 only
      D. 3 and 4 only

VIII. Maquet Servo^i/Servo^s Ventilator Systems

Upon completion of this section, you will be able to:
1. List the modes of ventilation available on the Maquet Servo^i and Servo^s.
2. Describe the alarms available on the Maquet Servo^i and Servo^s.
3. Identify the extended monitoring features on the Maquet Servo^i and Servo^s.
4. Describe the use of NAVA.
5. Compare the differences between the adult and neo-natal modes of ventilation.

ACHIEVING THE OBJECTIVES

1. List the modes of ventilation available on the Maquet Servo^i and Servo^s. (IIA6a)

1A. Which modes available on the Maquet Servo^i are controlled ventilation modes and offer full ventilatory support?

_____

_____

_____

1B. Which modes available on the Maquet Servo^i are considered supported ventilation modes?

_____

_____

1C. Which modes available on the Maquet Servo^i are considered spontaneous ventilation modes?

_____

_____

1D. Which modes available on the Maquet Servo^i are considered combined ventilation modes?

_____

_____

_____

2. Describe the alarms available on the Maquet Servo^i and Servo^s. (IIA6a)

2A. What are the three categories of alarms on the Maquet Servo^i?

_____

_____

_____

2B. What alarms are available on the Maquet Servo^i?

_____

_____

_____

2C. Explain the two ways that alarms may be set on the Maquet Servo^i?

_____

_____

_____

_____

_____

_____

_____

2D. How does the AUTOSET determine the alarm limits?

_____

_____

_____

_____

3. Identify the extended monitoring features on the Maquet Servo^i and Servo^s. (IIA6a)

3A. How is airway resistance displayed?

_____

_____

3B. What does the P_{01} indicate?

_____

_____

_____

_____

4. Describe the use of NAVA. (IIA6a)

4A. How does the NAVA option function?

_____

_____

4B. What does the patient require in order to use the NAVA option?

_____

_____

4C. What is the purpose of NAVA?

_____

_____

5. Compare the differences between adult and neonatal modes of ventilation. (IIA6a)

Refer to Figure 13-6 to answer Questions 5A and 5B.

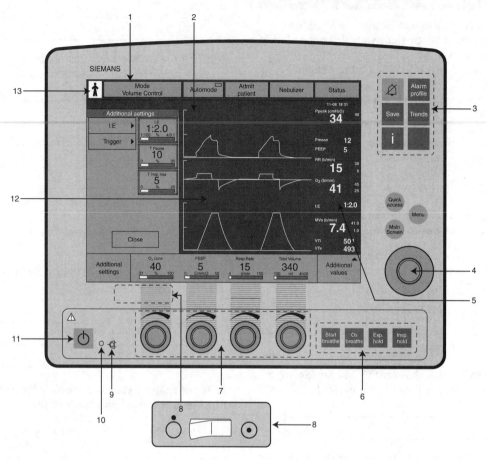

FIGURE 13-6
(Courtesy Maquet Incorporated, Bridgewater, NJ)

5A. Which of the Maquet Servo ventilators are able to provide neonatal ventilation?

_____

_____

5B. What modes of ventilation are available for neonatal ventilation?

_____

_____

_____

_____

Think About This:

What are the advantages of having a ventilator that does both NIV and invasive ventilation?

NATIONAL BOARD FOR RESPIRATORY CARE (NBRC)–TYPE QUESTIONS
MAQUET SERVO^i/SERVO^s

1. Which of the following statements is true concerning the Maquet Servo^i ventilator?
   A. The Servo^i cannot be adapted to use helium-oxygen (heliox).
   B. The ventilator can be adapted to be compatible with magnetic resonance imaging (MRI).
   C. Upgrading the unit requires a new central processing unit.
   D. AutoFlow facilitates weaning by allowing patient breath control.

2. While a Maquet Servo^i is operating in the PC mode, the low minute volume alarm becomes active. A patient assessment reveals bilateral inspiratory and expiratory wheezing. Which of the following represents the most-appropriate action for the respiratory therapist to take?
   A. Change to the VC mode.
   B. Increase the inspiratory cycle off setting.
   C. Decrease the low minute volume alarm.
   D. Administer a beta adrenergic bronchodilator.

3. When neurally adjusted ventilatory assist (NAVA) is in use, how/when is inspiration triggered?
   A. When the bias flow is reduced by 0.01 L/s.
   B. When pressure is reduced by 0.04 cm H_2O.
   C. By setting the cm H_2O/microvolts from 1 to 30.
   D. By setting the volume trigger to minimum.

4. All of the following are non-adjustable alarms on the Maquet Servo^i/Servo^s ventilators EXCEPT
   A. High continuous pressure
   B. O_2 concentration
   C. Gas supply
   D. High end-expiratory pressure

5. The Maquet Servo^s can operate in all of the following hospital areas or situations EXCEPT:
   1. Neonatal Intensive Care Unit
   2. During in-hospital transfers
   3. During MRI
   4. Pediatric Intensive Care Unit
      A. 1 only
      B. 1 and 3 only
      C. 2 and 4 only
      D. 3 and 4 only

173

Infant and Pediatric Devices

1. Systematically review continuous positive airway pressure (CPAP) delivery devices and ventilators used in the treatment of infant and pediatric patients.
2. List the various modes of ventilatory support provided by infant and pediatric ventilators.
3. Calculate the approximate tidal volume (V_T) delivered by a typical infant ventilator when given flow rate and inspiration time (T_I).
4. Describe the controls, monitors, alarms, and safety systems found on infant and pediatric ventilators.
5. Discuss precautions and key troubleshooting points for nasal CPAP devices and neonatal and pediatric ventilators.

"There is always one moment in childhood when the door opens and lets the future in."
Deepak Chopra

1. Systematically review CPAP delivery devices and ventilators used in the treatment of infant and pediatric patients. (IIA2, IIA6a, IIA6b, IIA6c)

1A. Identify the freestanding systems that are currently available for the delivery of CPAP.

_____

_____

_____

_____

1B. List the interfaces used to deliver nasal CPAP.

_____

_____

_____

_____

1C. What factors dictate which type of CPAP system and interface used in a facility?

_____

_____

_____

1D. Differentiate between CareFusion's Air*Life* Infant nCPAP System and Infant Flow SiPAP System.

_____

_____

_____

_____

1E. Why is the Fisher & Paykel Bubble CPAP System considered to be one of the most complicated systems on the market today?

_____

_____

_____

_____

1F. What is the significance of the differences in flow generators between CareFusion's Air*Life* Infant nCPAP System and Hamilton Medical's ARABELLA system?

_____

_____

_____

_____

1G. List the ventilators specifically designed for use in infants.

_____

_____

_____

_____

1H. Traditionally, infant ventilators were capable of providing _____ and _____ exclusively.

1I. What factors have allowed clinicians to apply additional modes during ventilation of infants today?

_____

_____

_____

_____

1J. _____ continues to be the most widely used mode in the ventilation of premature infants and infants of very low birth weight.

_____

_____

_____

1K. Describe time-cycled pressure-limited ventilation.

_____

_____

_____

_____

1L. Identify the two types of high-frequency ventilators used for infants and children.

_____

_____

1M. Bunnell's Life Pulse High Frequency "Jet" Ventilator (HFJV) is indicated for patients with

_____

_____

_____

_____

1N. Discuss the two methods of applying high-frequency jet ventilation by means of Bunnell's Life Pulse HFJV.

_____

_____

_____

_____

_____

1O. What is the difference between CareFusion's 3100A and 3100B High Frequency Oscillatory Ventilators?

_____

_____

_____

1P. Identify newer-generation general use ventilators that are capable of ventilating infants.

_____

_____

_____

_____

1Q. What types of flow sensors are recommended for the three available models of the CareFusion AVEA ventilator for infants weighing less than 5 kg?

_____

_____

_____

_____

1R. Dräger Evita XL

(1) What enables this ventilator's use in infants weighing less than 3 kg?

_____

_____

_____

_____

(2) What are the specifications of the NeoFlow sensor?

_____

_____

_____

_____

1S. Maquet Servo[i]

(1) What type of flow sensor is used with this ventilator for infants?

_____

_____

_____

_____

(2) What are the specifications of the flow sensor?

_____

_____

_____

_____

1T. Covidien Puritan Bennett (PB) 840

(1) What option makes this ventilator compatible with infant use?

_____

_____

_____

_____

(2) What else must be added to the ventilator to make it compatible with infant use?

_____

_____

_____

_____

Think About This:

What are the differences between the United States and Europe in terms of electrical voltage?

2. List the modes of ventilatory support provided by various infant and pediatric ventilators. (IIA6a)

	Device	Modes of ventilation
2A.	CareFusion V.I.P. Bird Infant/Pediatric Ventilator	
2B.	CareFusion V.I.P. Sterling and Gold Infant/Pediatric Ventilators	
2C.	Dräger Babylog 8000 infant ventilator	
2D.	Dräger Babylog 8000 plus infant ventilator	
2E.	CareFusion AVEA ventilator (for infant/pediatric use)	
2F.	Dräger Evita XL ventilator (for infant/pediatric use)	
2G.	Maquet Servo^i ventilator (for infant/pediatric use)	
2H.	Covidien PB 840 ventilator (for infant/pediatric use)	

Think About This:

What are the advantages and disadvantages of having one type of ventilator that can be used with patients of all ages (newborns, children, and adults)?

3. Calculate the approximate V_T delivered by a typical infant ventilator when given flow rate and T_I. (IIID2b)

Fill in the blanks in the following table:

	T_I (sec)	Flow (L/min)	V_T (mL)	Calculations
3A.	0.4	12		
3B.	0.5	10		
3C.	0.6	8		
3D.	0.75	15		
3E.		10	25	
3F.		8	10	
3G.	0.45		8	

Think About This:

Which is more accurate: calculating the V_T or measuring the volume with a pneumotachometer?

177

4. Describe the controls, monitors, alarm, and safety systems found on infant and pediatric ventilators. (IIA6a, IIA6b, IIA6c)

4A. CareFusion V.I.P. Bird (Figure 14-1):

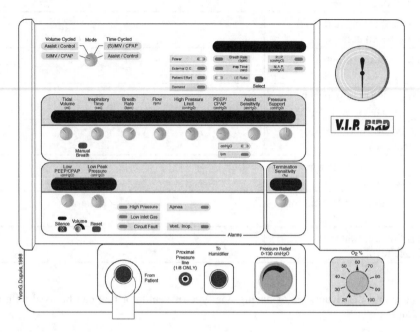

FIGURE 14-1
(Courtesy Yvon Dupuis.)

(1) What is the location of the mode selector, and how are the modes grouped?

_____

(2) What alarms are included in the alarm section on this ventilator's front panel?

_____

_____

(3) What additional safety feature is incorporated into this ventilator, and where is its control located?

_____

_____

(4) Explain the function of termination sensitivity.

_____

_____

(5) What happens to the breath when the inspiratory flow fails to decrease to the termination sensitivity set percentage?

_____

(6) Which control knob on this ventilator will set flow sensitivity?

_____

(7) When and how does leak compensation operate on this ventilator?

_____

_____

_____

(8) What variables does the CareFusion Bird Partner IIi Volume Monitor measure and display?

_____

_____

_____

(9) How can a continuous artificial airway leak be detected within the circuit of this ventilator?

_____

_____

4B. CareFusion V.I.P. Sterling and Gold Infant/Pediatric Ventilators (Figure 14-2):

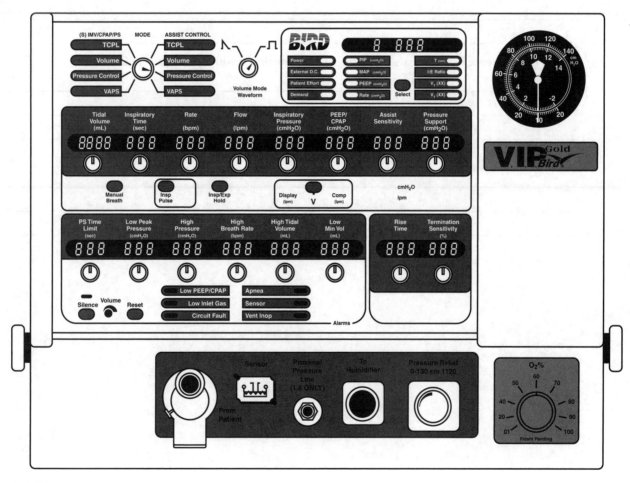

FIGURE 14-2
(Courtesy CareFusion VIASYS Healthcare, Critical Care Division, Palm Springs, California.)

(1) What is the location of the "Mode Select" switch, and how are the modes grouped?

_____

(2) Which flow waveforms are available during volume-controlled breaths?

_____

(3) How is the apnea interval determined and set?

_____

_____

_____

_____

_____

(4) What is rise time, and where is the control located on the Gold model?

_____

_____

_____

(5) What is the difference between assist sensitivity and termination sensitivity on this ventilator?

_____

_____

_____

(6) How is the bias flow adjusted on this ventilator?

_____

_____

_____

4C. Dräger Babylog 8000 Infant Ventilator (Figure 14-3):

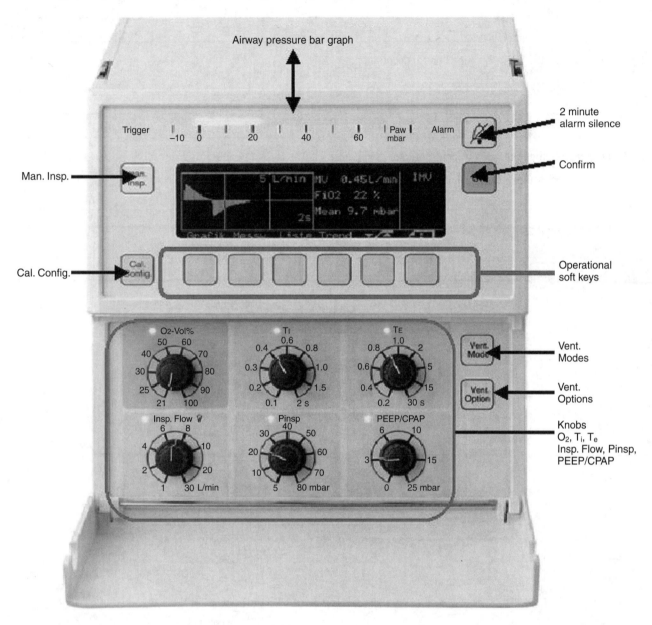

FIGURE 14-3
(Courtesy Dräger Medical AG & Co, Lübeck, Germany.)

(1) What controls does the rotary dial panel contain?

_____

_____

(2) What is the function of the soft keys?

_____

(3) How are alarms silenced and reset on this ventilator?

_____

_____

(4) Which alarms are set automatically by the ventilator, and what are their settings?

_____

_____

(5) How are the alarms grouped on this ventilator?

_____

_____

_____

4D. Dräger Babylog 8000 plus Infant Ventilator (see Figure 14-3):

(1) What does the "plus" term in the name of the ventilator indicate?

_____

(2) How are the monitoring parameters accessed on this ventilator?

_____

4E. Bunnell Life Pulse HFJV (Figure 14-4):

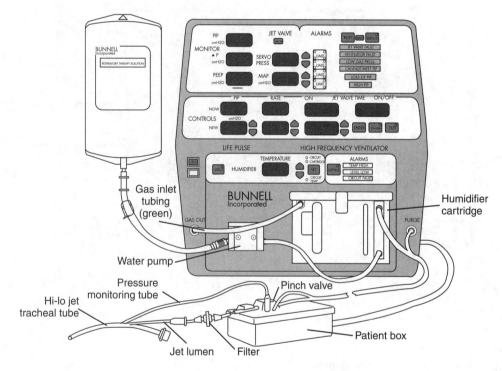

FIGURE 14-4
(Courtesy Bunnell Incorporated, Salt Lake City, Utah.)

(1) What parameters can be adjusted in the controls area on the front panel?

_____

(2) What does the jet valve time "On/Off" button represent?

_____

(3) What three buttons are located on the lower right portion of the controls area, and what are their functions?

_____

_____

_____

(4) List and explain the five parameters that are displayed in the monitor area.

    (a) _____

    (b) _____

    (c) _____

    (d) _____

    (e) _____

(5) List and explain the alarms located in the alarms area.

_____

_____

_____

_____

_____

_____

_____

_____

(6) What three buttons are located in the upper right corner of the alarms area? What functions do they serve?

    (a) _____

    (b) _____

    (c) _____

4F. CareFusion 3100A High Frequency Oscillatory Ventilator (Figure 14-5):

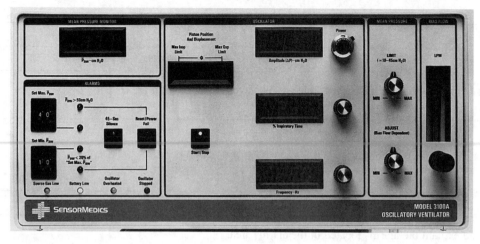

FIGURE 14-5
(Courtesy CareFusion VIASYS Healthcare, Critical Care Division, Palm Springs, California.)

(1) Describe the function of the flowmeter located on the right side of the front panel.

_____

_____

(2) What are the functions of the mean pressure "Adjust" and "Limit" controls?

_____

_____

_____

_____

_____

(3) Where is the mean airway pressure displayed?

_____

_____

(4) Describe the function of each control and display in the oscillator section.

_____

_____

_____

_____

_____

_____

_____

_____

_____

_____

_____

_____

_____

_____

(5) Where is the "On/Off" switch located?

_____

_____

(6) Describe the two switches in the alarms area.

_____

_____

_____

_____

_____

(7) What is the difference among the following alarms: "Set Max $\bar{P}_{aw}$," "Set Min $\bar{P}_{aw}$," "$\bar{P}_{aw} > 50$ cm H$_2$O," and "$\bar{P}_{aw} < 20\%$ of Set Max $\bar{P}_{aw}$"?

_____

_____

_____

_____

_____

_____

_____

_____

_____

_____

_____

_____

_____

_____

_____

_____

(8) What happens to the ventilator if electrical power is interrupted and then restored?

_____

_____

_____

_____

(9) If gas pressure fell to below 30 pound-force per square inch gauge (psig), which alarm would become visible?

_____

_____

(10) At what temperature will the yellow "oscillator overheated" light-emitting diode (LED) become visible?

_____

(11) What is the function of the yellow "battery low" LED?

_____

4G. CareFusion 3100B High Frequency Oscillatory Ventilator (see Figure 14-5):

(1) What controls on the 3100A model have been eliminated from the 3100B model?

_____

_____

(2) What are the differences between the alarm limits and function of the 3100B model and those of the 3100A model?

_____

_____

_____

_____

_____

(3) How does the bias flow control differ on the 3100B model?

_____

_____

Think About This:

What types of ventilators are used with very small animals?

185

5. Discuss precautions and key troubleshooting points for nasal CPAP devices and neonatal and pediatric ventilators. (IIA2, IIA6a, IIA6c)

5A. CareFusion's Infant Flow nCPAP System, Air*Life* Infant nCPAP System Driver, and Infant Flow SiPAP system and Fisher & Paykel's Bubble CPAP System:

(1) What are the most likely causes of leaks in any CPAP system?

_____

_____

(2) What may cause skin irritation and patient discomfort?

_____

_____

(3) If the rims of a patient's nostrils are blanched, the cause is probably

_____ .

(4) What can be done to restore CPAP if the CPAP system is not maintaining the set pressure because the infant's mouth is open?

_____

_____

5B. CareFusion V.I.P. Bird Infant/Pediatric Ventilator:

(1) In the assist/control time-cycled mode, the ventilator's "termination %" setting is flashing. What does this indicate, and what could be the cause?

_____

_____

_____

_____

(2) What can be done to stop self-triggering when the ventilator is in the volume-cycled synchronized intermittent mandatory ventilation mode?

_____

_____

_____

_____

5C. CareFusion V.I.P. Bird Sterling and Gold Infant/Pediatric Ventilators:

(1) How can a patient being ventilated with a V.I.P. Bird Gold Ventilator be checked with regard to the presence of intrinsic positive end-expiratory pressure (auto-PEEP)?

_____

_____

_____

_____

_____

5D. Dräger Babylog 8000 and 8000 plus Infant Ventilators:

(1) What is the likely cause of inaccurate minute ventilation monitoring?

_____

_____

_____

(2) What precautions should be taken when the volume guarantee mode is used on the 8000 plus ventilator?

_____

_____

_____

_____

5E. Bunnell Life Pulse HFJV:

(1) List four possible causes of a decrease in servo pressure.

_____

_____

_____

(2) List four possible causes of the "cannot meet PIP" (peak inspiratory pressure) alarm.

_____

_____

_____

(3) What may happen if the "Enter" button for new parameters is pressed before the patient circuit is connected to the patient?

_____

_____

5F. CareFusion 3100A High Frequency Oscillatory Ventilator:

(1) List two alarm situations that would cause the oscillator to stop.

_____

_____

(2) What immediate action should be taken if the oscillator stops?

_____

_____

(3) During operation, the piston position is noted to have moved toward the maximum inspiratory limit. What action should be taken?

_____

_____

(4) What could be the cause of the "Set Min $\overline{P}_{aw}$" alarm?

_____

_____

5G. CareFusion 3100B High Frequency Oscillatory Ventilator:

(1) List three possible causes for the "$\overline{P}_{aw}$ Set Max" alarm to go on.

_____

_____

_____

(2) What procedure should be followed after a temporary disconnection, such as for routine suctioning?

_____

_____

_____

_____

5H. CareFusion AVEA ventilator for infant/pediatric use:

Volumes that are consistently lower than set are being delivered to a pediatric patient, and there is no significant leakage around the endotracheal tube. What is the possible cause of this problem?

_____

_____

5I. Dräger Evita XL Ventilator for infant/pediatric use:

(1) Before the NeoFlow sensor is placed into the circuit, what needs to be done to the sensor?

_____

_____

(2) What happens to the ventilator if the neonatal flow sensor becomes partially occluded with water or secretions?

_____

_____

_____

_____

_____

_____

_____

5J. Maquet Servo^i Ventilator for neonatal and pediatric use:

(1) What action should be taken when there is an audible and visual high-priority alarm with the message "Ventilating in Back-up Mode"?

_____

_____

_____

_____

(2) What could cause the ventilator to automatically increase the set flow rate during the use of nasal CPAP?

_____

_____

_____

_____

5K. Covidien PB 840 Ventilator for infant/pediatric use:

(1) Why are low-compliance humidifiers most suitable for pediatric/neonatal use?

_____

_____

(2) Why is it necessary to run a short self-test when the ventilator is reset for neonatal use?

_____

_____

_____

_____

Think About This:

What are your thoughts about the advantages and disadvantages of a respiratory care department having separate infant ventilators versus having general-use ventilators with infant/pediatric capabilities?

NATIONAL BOARD FOR RESPIRATORY CARE (NBRC)–TYPE QUESTIONS

1. CareFusion's 3100A and 3100B High Frequency Oscillatory Ventilators have what type of internal mechanism?
   A. Pinch valves
   B. Rotary drive piston
   C. Linear drive piston
   D. Proportional solenoid valves

2. Lowering the frequency setting on CareFusion's 3100A or 3100B High Frequency Oscillatory Ventilator will cause which of the following?
   A. Increase in volume
   B. Decrease in volume
   C. Decrease in piston travel time
   D. Change in percentage of T_I

3. Which of the following infant ventilators requires a triple-lumen, uncuffed endotracheal tube?
   A. CareFusion V.I.P. Bird
   B. Dräger Babylog 8000 plus
   C. Bunnell Life Pulse HFJV
   D. CareFusion 3100A High Frequency Oscillatory Ventilator

4. During a time-cycled, pressure-limited breath with the CareFusion V.I.P. Bird Gold model, a minimum V_T may be guaranteed by an automatic increase in which of the following?
   A. Rise time
   B. Flow rate
   C. Inspiratory phase
   D. Inspiratory pressure

5. For a neonate who requires mechanical ventilation, a Dräger Babylog 8000 ventilator is being set up in the intermittent mandatory ventilation mode. Which combination of T_I and expiratory time (T_E) will provide a mandatory rate of 45 breaths/min with a ratio of T_I to T_E of 1:3?
   A. 0.18 second, 0.55 second
   B. 0.33 second, 1.00 second
   C. 0.50 second, 1.50 second
   D. 0.75 second, 2.25 seconds

6. The CPAP device that can provide bi-level airway pressure for small infants is which of the following?
   A. Hamilton Medical ARABELLA system
   B. CareFusion Infant Flow SiPAP system
   C. CareFusion AirLife Infant nCPAP (nasal CPAP) System Driver
   D. Fisher & Paykel Bubble CPAP System

7. Calculate the maximum available V_T for time-triggered, pressure-limited, time-cycled ventilation when T_I is 0.5 second and the flow rate is set at 7 L/min.
   A. 35 mL
   B. 42 mL
   C. 58 mL
   D. 210 mL

8. Calculate the flow rate to deliver 4 mL/kg volume to a 1250-g neonate with a 0.75-second T_I.
   A. 0.003 L/min
   B. 0.4 L/min
   C. 3 L/min
   D. 4 L/min

9. Which mode on the Dräger Babylog 8000 plus ventilator should not be used when there is a significant positional endotracheal tube leak?
   A. CPAP
   B. Pressure-limited SiPAP
   C. Synchronized intermittent mandatory ventilation (SIMV) + volume guarantee
   D. Pressure-limited SIMV

10. A proximal flow sensor is used for neonatal ventilation in all the following ventilators except:
    A. Covidien PB 840
    B. CareFusion AVEA
    C. Dräger Evita XL
    D. Maquet Servo[i]

15 Transport, Home Care, and Noninvasive Ventilatory Devices

LEARNING OBJECTIVES

Upon completion of this chapter you will be able to:

1. Give the value in liters/minute of the logic flow for the patient-disconnect feature when the Airon pNeuton model A ventilator is in use.
2. Determine the length of time that elapses between a low-battery event and a ventilator-inoperative event with the Bio-Med Crossvent ventilator when there is a power loss.
3. State the value for the gas supply pressure that will result in a low–source pressure alarm when the Bio-Med Crossvent 3+ ventilator is in use.
4. Describe the operating features, alarms, and parameter ranges of the following ventilators: Bio-Med Crossvent, Bio-Med MVP-10, Impact 731 EMV+, CareFusion Pulmonetic Systems LTV 1200, Newport HT70, and CareFusion ReVel.
5. Describe the affect of the oxygen flow on oxygen delivery in the Dräger Oxylog 3000 Plus ventilator.
6. Explain the function of the apnea alarm on the Impact Uni-Vent 750 ventilator.
7. Provide the value for logic gas consumption on the Impact Uni-Vent Eagle 754 ventilator.
8. State the liter flow necessary to operate the internal logic of the Percussionaire Bronchotron TXP ventilator.
9. Review the function of the Smiths Medical Pneupac ventiPAC ventilator's low-pressure "eyeball" alarm.
10. Discuss the ability of the Newport HT50 ventilator to provide enriched oxygen delivery.
11. Describe the adjustment of the positive end-expiratory pressure/continuous positive airway pressure (PEEP/CPAP) control on the Newport HT50 ventilator.
12. Give the amount of time that the Newport HT70 ventilator's secondary backup battery maintains operation without interruption when the main Power Pac battery is depleted.
13. Tell how long the internal ventilator battery will operate on the CareFusion ReVel ventilator.
14. Name the two operator-adjustable alarms on the Respironics BiPAP Focus ventilator.
15. Discuss the optional average volume assured pressure support (AVAPS) mode with the Respironics V60 ventilator.
16. Give the patient size limit for the Respironics Synchrony ventilator.
17. List the alarms available on the Covidien-Puritan Bennett GoodKnight 425 ventilator.
18. List the adjustable level of PEEP available with the CareFusion ResMed Stellar 100 ventilator.

"Life's a voyage that's homeward bound."
Herman Melville

ACHIEVING THE OBJECTIVES

1. Give the value in liters/minute of the logic flow for the patient-disconnect feature when the Airon pNeuton model A ventilator is in use. (IIA6a, IIA6b, III.I3a, III.I3b)

1A. Why does the alarm system require gas flow to operate?

_____

1B. How much gas is used by the Airon pNeuton model A ventilator for its pneumatically operated control system?

_____

Think About This:

Why can a pneumatically operated ventilator be used during magnetic resonance imaging?

2. Determine the length of time that elapses between a low-battery event and a ventilator-inoperative event with the Bio-Med Crossvent Ventilator when there is a power loss. (IIA6a, IIA6b, III.I3a, III.I3b)

2A. What is the operational time of a fully charged direct-current battery for the Bio-Med Crossvent ventilator?

_____

2B. How much remaining time does the direct-current battery have when the "Low Battery, Connect External Power" message is displayed on the liquid-crystal graph screen?

_____

Think About This:

Why should most ventilators be plugged in even if they are not being used?

3. State the value for the gas supply pressure that will result in a low–source pressure alarm when the Bio-Med Crossvent 3+ ventilator is in use. (IIA6a, IIA6b, III.I3a, III.I3b)

3A. The Bio-Med Crossvent 3+ ventilator requires how much gas pressure to ensure adequate gas flow to the patient?

_____

3B. What source gas pressure will activate a low–source pressure alarm?

_____

Think About This:

What sizes of oxygen cylinders are used during flight transports?

4. Describe the operating features, alarms, and ventilator parameter ranges of the following ventilators: (IIA6a, IIA6b, III.I3a, III.I3b)

- Bio-Med Crossvent
- Bio-Med MVP-10
- Impact 731 EMV+
- CareFusion Pulmonetic Systems LTV 1200
- Newport HT70
- CareFusion ReVel

4A. Complete the following table for the Bio-Med Crossvent 3+ ventilator:

Operating Features		Alarms		Parameters	
Population				Rate	
Designation				Tidal Volume	
Power Source				Inspiratory Time	
Battery				Inspiration/Expiration (I/E) Ratio	
Modes				Flow Rate	
				Peak Pressure	
				PEEP/CPAP	
				Fraction of Inspired Oxygen (F_IO_2)	

4B. Complete the following table for the Bio-Med MVP-10 ventilator:

Operating Features			Alarms	Parameters	
Population				Rate	
Designation				Tidal Volume	
Power Source				Inspiratory Time	
Battery				I/E Ratio	
Modes				Flow Rate	
				Peak Pressure	
				PEEP/CPAP	
				F_IO_2	

4C. Complete the following table for the Impact 731 EMV+ ventilator:

Operating Features			Alarms	Parameters	
Population				Rate	
Designation				Tidal Volume	
Power Source				Inspiratory Time	
Battery				I/E Ratio	
Modes				Flow Rate	
				Peak Pressure	
				PEEP/CPAP	
				F_IO_2	

4D. Complete the following table for the CareFusion Pulmonetic Systems LTV 1200 ventilator:

Operating Features		Alarms	Parameters	
Population			Rate	
Designation			Tidal Volume	
Power Source			Inspiratory Time	
Battery			I/E Ratio	
Modes			Flow Rate	
			Peak Pressure	
			PEEP/CPAP	
			F_IO_2	

4E. Complete the following table for the Newport HT70 ventilator:

Operating Features		Alarms	Parameters	
Population			Rate	
Designation			Tidal Volume	
Power Source			Inspiratory Time	
Battery			I/E Ratio	
Modes			Flow Rate	
			Peak Pressure	
			PEEP/CPAP	
			F_IO_2	

4F. Complete the following table for the CareFusion ReVel ventilator:

Operating Features		Alarms	Parameters	
Population			Rate	
Designation			Tidal Volume	
Power Source			Inspiratory Time	
Battery			I/E Ratio	
Modes			Flow Rate	
			Peak Pressure	
			PEEP/CPAP	
			F_IO_2	

Think About This:
Which of these ventilators is best suited for a patient with a wheelchair?

5. Describe the effect of the oxygen flow on oxygen delivery by the Dräger Oxylog 3000 Plus ventilator. (IIA6a, IIA6b, III.I3a, III.I3b)

_____

_____

_____

_____

_____

_____

_____

_____

Think About This:
How can the Dräger Oxylog 3000 Plus ventilator ensure that the F_IO_2 is between 21% and 40%?

6. Explain the function of the apnea alarm on the Impact Uni-Vent 750 ventilator. (IIA6a, III.I3a, III.I3b)

6A. Explain the function of the apnea alarm on the Impact Uni-Vent 750 ventilator.

_____

_____

_____

_____

_____

_____

Think About This:
What are the advantages and disadvantages of automatic apnea alarm settings?

193

7. Provide the value for logic gas consumption on the Impact Uni-Vent Eagle 754 ventilator. (IIA6a, IIA6b, III.I3a, III.I3b)

_____

_____

_____

_____

Think About This:
What are the criteria to be included in the Strategic National Stockpile?

8. State the liter flow required to operate the internal logic of the Percussionaire Bronchotron TXP ventilator. (IIA6a, IIA6b, III.I3a, III.I3b)

_____

Think About This:
What types of patients would benefit from high-frequency ventilation during transport?

9. Review the function of the Smiths Medical Pneupac ventiPAC low-gas supply "eyeball" alarm. (IIA6a, IIA6b, III.I3a, III.I3b)

_____

_____

_____

_____

_____

Think About This:
How much gas supply should be available during a transport?

10. Discuss the ability of the Newport HT50 ventilator to provide enriched oxygen delivery. (IIIK1, IIIK9)

10A. Describe the function of the air–oxygen entrainment mixer.

_____

_____

_____

10B. How does the oxygen-blending bag kit operate?

_____

_____

_____

_____

Think About This:
Which oxygen-delivery system is most appropriate for the hospital and which for the home?

11. Describe the adjustment of the PEEP/CPAP control on the Newport HT50 ventilator. (IIIK1, IIIK9)

11A. What happens to the sensitivity setting when PEEP is initiated?

_____

11B. What is the range of PEEP available on the Newport HT50 ventilator?

_____

11C. During pressure-control ventilation with PEEP, what is the maximum amount of PEEP that can be set?

_____

Think About This:
Can auto-PEEP occur during home ventilation?

12. Give the amount of time the Newport HT70 ventilator's secondary backup battery maintains operation without interruption when the main Power Pac battery is depleted. (IIIK1, IIIK9)

_____

13. State how long the internal ventilator battery will operate on the Pulmonetic Systems LTV 800 ventilator. (IIIK1, IIIK9)

_____

Think About This:
Which transport or home care ventilator has the battery with the longest operation time?

14. Name the two operator-adjustable alarms on the Respironics BiPAP Focus ventilator. (IIIK1, IIIK9)

_____

_____

Think About This:
It is estimated that more than 12 million American adults have sleep apnea (National Heart, Lung, and Blood Institute).

15. Discuss the optional AVAPS mode with the Respironics V60 ventilator. (IIIK1, IIIK9)

_____

_____

_____

_____

_____

_____

Think About This:

Other than people with sleep apnea, what other patients could benefit from BiPAP?

16. Give the patient size limit for the Respironics Synchrony ventilator. (IIIK1, IIIK9)

_____

_____

Think About This:

Is it age or weight that dictates whether a person is considered a pediatric patient or an adult patient?

17. List the alarms available on the Covidien-Puritan Bennett GoodKnight 425 ventilator. (IIIK1, IIIK9)

_____

_____

18. List the adjustable level of PEEP available with the CareFusion ResMed Stellar 100. (IIIK1, IIIK9)

_____

Think About This:

Getting used to BiPAP or CPAP is like training for an athletic event: the patient needs to work up to it.

Chapter **15** **Transport, Home Care, and Noninvasive Ventilatory Devices**

NATIONAL BOARD FOR RESPIRATORY CARE (NBRC)–TYPE QUESTIONS

1. Transport ventilators' capabilities should include all *except* which of the following?
   A. Ability to operate in extreme temperatures
   B. Easily recognizable controls
   C. A full range of modes from which to choose
   D. Sufficient shielding

2. The transport ventilator that can operate up to an altitude of 15,000 feet is
   A. Airon pNeuton model A
   B. Bio-Med Crossvent
   C. Dräger Oxylog 3000 Plus
   D. Smiths Medical Pneupac ventiPAC

3. A 2-kg premature newborn requires transport to a level 3 neonatal unit. The ventilator that needs to be used for this transport is which of the following?
   A. Bio-Med MVP-10
   B. Dräger Oxylog 3000 Plus
   C. Impact Uni-Vent 750
   D. Impact Uni-Vent Eagle 754

4. During a transport in which the patient is using a Smiths Medical Pneupac ventiPAC ventilator, the respiratory therapist notices the eyeball indicator turning red. The most appropriate action to take at this time is which of the following?
   A. Suction the patient's airway immediately.
   B. Change out the gas supply to the ventilator.
   C. Analyze the oxygen concentration being delivered.
   D. Remove the patient from the ventilator and manually ventilate.

5. The ventilators that can be used invasively or noninvasively in the home are which of the following?
   (1) Puritan Bennett LP10
   (2) Pulmonetic Systems LTV 800
   (3) Newport HT70
   (4) Puritan Bennett GoodKnight 425
   A. 1 and 2 only
   B. 2 and 3 only
   C. 3 and 4 only
   D. 1 and 4 only

6. A 42-year-old male trauma victim who requires magnetic resonance imaging (MRI) can be transported with which of the following?
   (1) Pulmonetic Systems LTV 800
   (2) Airon pNeuton model A
   (3) Impact Uni-Vent 750
   (4) Bio-Med MVP-10
   A. 1 only
   B. 1 and 2 only
   C. 2 and 3 only
   D. 2 and 4 only

7. The transport ventilator that can deliver respiratory rates upto 700 breaths/min is which of the following?
   A. Airon pNeuton model A
   B. Bio-Med Crossvent
   C. Smiths Medical Pneupac ventiPAC
   D. Percussionaire Bronchotron TXP

8. A transport ventilator that provides end-tidal CO_2 monitoring is the
   A. Bio-Med Crossvent
   B. Dräger Oxylog 3000 Plus
   C. Impact Uni-Vent 750
   D. CareFusion LTV 1000

9. During a patient transport with the Bio-Med Crossvent, the alarm menu begins to flash "Low Battery, Connect External Power" on the liquid-crystal graph screen. How much internal battery time is left?
   A. 5 minutes
   B. 10 minutes
   C. 15 minutes
   D. 20 minutes

10. The F_IO_2 delivery of the Impact Uni-Vent 750 is dependent on which of the following?
    (1) Air/mix switch setting
    (2) The gas source being used
    (3) Attachment of the blending bag kit
    (4) Flow rate of the oxygen bleed into the system
    A. 1 only
    B. 2 only
    C. 3 and 4 only
    D. 1 and 4 only